OXFORD MEDICAL PUBLICATIONS

Cystic Fibrosis

THE FACTS

Cystic Fibrosis

THE FACTS

ANN HARRIS
Lecturer in Molecular Biology
Guy's Hospital Medical School

and

MAURICE SUPER
Consultant Clinical Geneticist, Royal
Manchester Children's Hospital

OXFORD   NEW YORK   TOKYO
OXFORD UNIVERSITY PRESS
1987

Oxford University Press, Walton Street, Oxford OX2 6DP
Oxford New York Toronto
Delhi Bombay Calcutta Madras Karachi
Petaling Jaya Singapore Hong Kong Tokyo
Nairobi Dar es Salaam Cape Town
Melbourne Auckland
and associated companies in
Beirut Berlin Ibadan Nicosia

Oxford is a trade mark of Oxford University Press

Published in the United States
by Oxford University Press, New York

© Ann Harris and Maurice Super, 1987

All rights reserved. No part of this publication may be reproduced,
stored in a retrieval system, or transmitted, in any form or by any means,
electronic, mechanical, photocopying, recording, or otherwise, without
the prior permission of Oxford University Press

British Library Cataloguing in Publication Data
Harris, Ann
Cystic fibrosis: the facts.—(The Facts)
1. Cystic fibrosis
I. Title   II. Super, Maurice   III. Series
616.3'7   RC858.C95
ISBN 0-19-261462-2

Set by
Katerprint Typesetting Services, Oxford
Printed in Great Britain by
Richard Clay Ltd
Bungay, Suffolk

2 1858/616.37

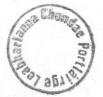

Acknowledgements

The authors would like to thank Mrs Georgina Briody, Miss Lynette Noble, and Miss Despina Savva for help with preparation of the manuscript and figures.

We are most grateful to Dr Duncan Matthew and Mrs Doris MacGlashan for helpful criticism of the manuscript and Miss Elizabeth Manners for proof-reading.

Figure 3 was provided by Dr R. Fraser Williams and Fig. 12 by the cytogenetics department of the Paediatric Research Unit, Guy's Hospital.

A.H. would like to thank Professor Paul E. Polani, who introduced her to the subject, and the Winston Churchill Memorial Trust for generous support.

M.S. thanks Dr Garry Hambleton for helpful discussions.

Contents

Introduction: living with cystic fibrosis

The needs of a child with cystic fibrosis (CF) change with age, but are generally much greater than those of a healthy child. Early on, the parents must help with regular physiotherapy, give medication, and provide a special diet. They have to learn to tolerate a certain amount of illness in the child and to know when medical help or advice is needed. It is very easy for one or other parent, often the father, to 'opt out' of such decisions and to participate little in the child's treatment. The efficient CF clinic, operating an 'open door' policy, can help to make both parents part of the team and may defuse many of the inherent tensions associated with CF. Even so, both parents and children have psychological ups and downs, sometimes feeling optimistic about the long-term outlook, sometimes pessimistic. The age at which a relative died of CF, or the death of a friend attending the CF clinic, may provide crisis points. Some adolescent rebellion against daily treatment may have its roots in depression. Some studies have shown that mothers of CF children become depressed from time to time, perhaps because they carry the main family burden of the illness.

For schoolchildren a persistent cough may be embarrassing and disrupt the class. Strong-smelling flatus (breaking of wind) or bulkiness of stools can be even more of a problem. Luckily with present-day special diets and improvements in the strength and quality of pancreatic supplements, fewer patients nowadays have this problem. The school may need to be asked to provide a special diet. Pamphlets for teachers (e.g. 'A child with cystic fibrosis in your class', prepared by the CF Trust) may help the child's problems to be dealt with sympathetically, as may visits to the school by the CF nurse or dietician. Illness may result in the loss of many school-

1

days. Generally the child will be well enough to do at least some work at home, and most children with CF manage to keep up remarkably well. As far as possible special schools for the physically disabled are to be avoided. Similarly, one tries to avoid home tutors as long-term substitutes for school attendance.

As the child becomes older the parents may find the physiotherapy physically taxing. The forced expiration technique described in the chapter on management may liberate them and provide the child with greater independence.

Adolescence brings its own problems. Differences in height and weight may become more marked, and a delayed growth spurt can mean that CF children may lag behind other children of the same age. In the less well nourished there may also be significant delay in sexual maturation. Adolescent rebellion may result in loss of co-operation in taking medicines, having physiotherapy, and controlling diet. At about 16 years of age, we believe there is benefit in transferring to the adult CF clinic if one exists. Being allowed to 'grow up' in this way may provide the stimulus to vigorous treatment once more.

In this competitive day and age adult CF sufferers may have to cope with unemployment, though many manage remarkably well in a wide variety of careers. Certain very physical occupations are closed to all but the most mildly affected. Affected men will have to cope with the almost invariable sterility (though not impotence), and women need to remember the possible very adverse effect on health that a pregnancy may have, the physical hard work involved in caring for an infant, and the 1 in 50 or so risk they run of having an affected child.

LIVING WITH CYSTIC FIBROSIS

The following are the comments of members of two different families who live daily with the problems of cystic fibrosis.

Introduction: living with cystic fibrosis

First, David aged 13, diagnosed as having CF at nine weeks.
Being a child with CF isn't terrible, but it can be a bit of a pain in
the neck. We try to be as normal as possible, but it can be quite
difficult, with all the work involved. Probably the worst thing is diet, children with CF find it difficult
to put on weight. All the things normal children eat are forbidden
to us, like crisps, chocolate, and anything else containing a lot of
fat. We are stuck on a low-fat diet and most of our food is grilled
or fried in a special low-fat oil called MCT oil.
Another thing is physio. This has to be done twice per day, or if
I have a cold or something like that, as many times as it needs to be
cleared out. Physio isn't much fun if I'm in someone else's house
watching videos or listening to records, because I always have to
come home that bit sooner. School is quite normal. I go to an
ordinary school and do everything that other children do. I take a
packed lunch because most of the school meals are fried. I have a
lot of friends and get on with nearly everyone. You do get the odd
wisecrack about your weight, but you either ignore them or give
them a mouthful.
Every so often, I have to go into hospital for 10 days, which can
be quite boring. In hospital, I am on intensive physio and i.v.
[intravenous] treatment. Hospital isn't that bad, but when I get
back to school I have quite a lot of work to copy up.
All together, CF is hard work, but it isn't as bad for me as it's
made out to be.

David's mother's thoughts follow:

Being a parent of a CF child can be a demanding and very
frustrating role. It affects you both mentally and physically. There
isn't a moment of the day when CF is not in your thoughts. A
routine has to be worked out, as everything revolves around these
children. When you are told that your child has CF it is devastat-
ing, and when someone's child is ill all the other parents feel it and
worry.
David is a very sensible and active 13-year-old, but he is susceptible to severe chest infections. If a cold is going around, he will
catch it, and his normally twice a day physio will have to be
stepped up, sometimes to every two hours, to keep on top of it. A
cold can make him quite ill. Needless to say, both parent and child
end up very tired and sometimes very argumentative. When David

3

comes in a bit late, he does not want his physio done, and I don't feel like doing it. It would be very easy to say 'let's leave it', but it doesn't work that way and it's got to be done properly.

School causes quite a big problem, as there is always someone in the classroom who has got some infection to pass around; this is a constant worry. We have fortunately got a very understanding school, and the teachers have come to comprehend just what is wrong with David. Many parents have great difficulties in this area and for the children it can be a distressing situation. Being called 'skinny' isn't funny. David is with a grand set of lads who help him a lot and don't mind his coughs. One of the most intensely worrying times is when David is admitted to hospital. Having lost one boy with CF I dread the words 'X-ray' and what the doctors will tell me, but always strength seems to come from somewhere.

A low-fat diet is essential, but can sometimes prove 'a bit of a pain'. I think that once in a while small treats have to be given.

A doctor once asked me if he should paint the blackest picture to the parents. The answer is yes. The parent has to realize from the very start just what the situation is — the importance of the physio and diet and the consequences if these are not done.

Both parents have to pull together, and it isn't always easy. CF can either make you drift apart or pull you closer together. We are very fortunate.

CF children need a lot of time and attention, more so when they are not very well, and the mental strain is terrible. Bitterness does sometimes creep into it and you ask yourself, 'Why me?'. The answer is simple — I tell myself I'm special and have been given a very special child to look after.

Next, the comments of three brothers, Adam, Matthew, and Dominic. Adam and Matthew have cystic fibrosis, while the eldest, Dominic, does not. Diagnoses were made at 11 months in Adam and at the age of one month in Matthew. Both affected boys have had nasal polyps removed and Matthew has had an abdominal operation for an obstruction of the lower intestine after the newborn period (meconium ileus equivalent; see Chapter 2).

Adam, aged 14. To me cystic fibrosis generally means a low fat diet, physiotherapy, antibiotics, and an amount of inconvenience.

4

Introduction: living with cystic fibrosis

I often find physiotherapy to be the most inconvenient. Usually school holidays cause problems as I cannot go without one of my parents coming along to do my physio. This may not seem much of a problem, but it prevents me having too much freedom.

Enzymes are no longer a problem for me. I used to mix four Pancrex capsules with 10 ml of liquid antibiotic, but now I just swallow two Pancrease capsules with each meal, which I find a lot more convenient. The low fat diet I can also cope with. It is also (I find) a very healthy diet. Cutting out fats, chocolates or greasy foods leaves me without spots or greasy skin. If by some amazing miracle I was cured tomorrow, I don't think that I would rush out and buy a bar of Cadbury's or a bag of chips. With me as healthy as I am now, who needs one?

Finally my chest complaints. These leave me with no troubles as I am regular full-back for my high school Rugby League team.

Dominic, aged 17. Living with two brothers who suffer from cystic fibrosis can sometimes be very hard, but most of the time it isn't really that bad. I have to get up very early in the morning, at about 7.00 a.m., to help in the kitchen while the boys are having their physiotherapy. I don't really mind doing this, as I have got so used to it over the past few years, although I sometimes get irritable and argumentative over the slightest things.

I sometimes, rather selfishly, think that having physiotherapy is an excuse to miss out on helping with jobs around the house, but I have to realize that it cannot be helped if my brothers have cystic fibrosis. As physiotherapy is such an important part of their treatment, holidays may be slightly spoiled, over time allowed for going out during the day and at night, as it takes about half an hour for physio. It doesn't spoil all our holidays though, as we sometimes go to Lourdes, in France, to allow the boys to bathe in the waters and to pray for a cure, as well as being tourists.

Most of the things I can have, they can't have, and so little arguments may begin, although I may argue over the things they get instead. Also, most of the time, I get on very well with my brothers, as they try to live normal lives, and I only hope that a cure for cystic fibrosis may soon come in the near future.

Overall, having to live with cystic fibrosis sufferers isn't really a big thing. We all manage to get on together as one big, happy family.

Matthew, aged 12. There are many different aspects to cystic fibrosis. Some are good, some are not so good. We usually get up at about 6.30 a.m. for our physiotherapy. That means going to bed earlier than normal, non-cystic children. It can be very inconvenient at times. For instance, last time I went on a camping holiday with the school, my dad had to come with me to do my physio which made me feel not as free to mess about as the others. I am on a strict low fat diet which sometimes 'gets me down'. Sometimes when I can't have some things, people feel sorry for me and maybe give me money or my favourite sweets. The medicines we take are not that bad. I suppose the taste just grows on us. Altogether though, cystic fibrosis is not that bad and there are people in the world who are much more ill than me.

These comments by family members provide certain insights. We were able to reassure David's mother that he and other children with CF are not unduly susceptible to the mild infections of the schoolroom and that his immune system would cope with them quite normally without their causing deterioration of his CF. Many parents of younger children with CF need this reassurance to help prevent them mollycoddling the child. In David's mother's case her general worry about his advanced illness depresses her from time to time. When depression occurs it is generally the mother who shows it. David is exasperated by being undersized and about his illness in general but not depressed.

In common with many older children with CF, Matthew, Adam and to a lesser extent David show denial of their disorder and its potential seriousness. This is a very common coping mechanism and is shared by many of the medical and paramedical members of the CF team. The latter need to be very positively orientated towards vigorous treatment but need to retain the insight that they may not always succeed.

Many of the psychological problems in CF spring from the unknown. It is difficult to face up to a disorder in which the long-term outlook for any individual may be impossible to predict. Some children go through a phase of repeated quite severe chest infections only to recover and stay well for

6

years. Others do not recover or suffer the effects of permanent lung damage. There is always the hope of a miracle
cure being discovered.

The infertility of males and the potential dangers of pregnancy in females contribute to only 10% of adult males
marrying and only 33% of adult females. This said, people
with CF do form lasting relationships.

The CF clinic, through the CF nurse, ward sister, physiotherapist, or dietician, plays a very important role in providing a listening ear and parents are encouraged to 'phone in
with their queries or worries. In the beginning this may act
as a crutch until self-confidence builds up. Life used to be
more restricted for CF children — with the new more powerful pancreatic enzymes dietary 'indiscretion' at a party is less
important. Perhaps full cream items still need to be avoided
but an extra Pancrease or two with the party food should
avoid stomach-ache or loose stools. Many children are now
allowed a normal diet. Lethargy is an important danger sign
and often signifies salt depletion. This occurs mainly but not
exclusively in hot weather. It is quite easy to control, if
thought of. Unexplained diarrhoea may signify a new chest
infection rather than a dietary problem. So may a change in
sputum colour, an increase in sputum or general irritability.
They should all be reported to the doctor.

Except for neglecting physiotherapy and other CF treatment there are very few absolute 'don'ts' in CF.

This sketched outline of CF is elaborated on in the subsequent chapters.

1

What is cystic fibrosis?

Cystic fibrosis is an inherited disease that has its main effects on the digestive system and the lungs. It is usually diagnosed soon after birth, and symptoms occur throughout life. Nowadays, thanks to improvements in dietary supplements and better treatment, most people with cystic fibrosis can lead a fairly normal life. However, they need a special diet and regular physiotherapy; they also tend to be prone to chest infections.

The name cystic fibrosis (CF) describes the changes that occur at an early age in the pancreas of CF patients. (The pancreas is a major organ in the body, manufacturing digestive enzymes and other important compounds). The part of the pancreas that produces digestive enzymes (proteins that digest food) is replaced by a characteristic fibrous scar tissue with fluid-filled spaces (cysts). Since the basic cause of the disease remains unknown, the name cystic fibrosis continues to be used for convenience.

Another common feature of CF is unusually sticky or viscid mucus secretions in the lungs and digestive system. In the lungs the presence of this viscid mucus makes chest infections more severe, while in the digestive system it may damage the pancreas. This viscid mucus is the origin of another common name for CF, mucoviscidosis.

Until the beginning of this century doctors did not recognize CF as a disease in its own right. The various symptoms of CF were merely seen as separate, unrelated infections. Part of the reason for this was that before the advent of antibiotics, chest infections (which are a major feature of CF) were common in many diseases. The first recognition of CF came through another feature of the disease, namely steatorrhoea. Steatorrhoea means literally 'fatty stools', and is a condition characterized by the passage of pale, bulky, smelly faeces. Thus in 1912 the London physician Archibald Garrod described the occurrence of steatorrhoea in several members of the same family. The description, with hindsight, was almost certainly of CF.

The next clear description of CF came from a Swiss paediatrician named Fanconi. He described children with cystic fibrosis in 1928 and again in 1936. He also distinguished CF from coeliac disease, a disease caused by an inability to digest wheat proteins that has some symptoms in common with CF. When the initial descriptions of CF were made, there was some controversy as to whether steatorrhoea and recurrent attacks of severe bronchitis constituted a separate disease (both symptoms were common to several diseases in the pre-antibiotic era). It was not until other chest and digestive system diseases (e.g. pneumonia and bacillary dysentery) became treatable that this controversy was resolved.

It was found that in some cases treatment of chest or gut infections was ineffective, or gave only temporary relief. The patients unaffected by treatment were identified as CF sufferers. Thus Fanconi, working in Zurich, and Dorothy Anderson in Baltimore, were proved correct in recognizing CF as a specific disorder. A paper by Dorothy Anderson in 1938 gave an almost complete account of the development of CF, and a further paper in 1946 advocated treatment of the disease with a high-calorie, high-protein, low-fat diet supplemented with pancreatin (extract of animal pancreas). In 1948 Anderson and her co-worker Di'Santagnese confirmed another characteristic of the disease. They showed that CF patients are particularly prone to chest infections caused by *Staphylococcus* bacteria.

In 1952 there was a heatwave in New York. Perceptive physicians noted that the majority of children brought to casualty departments with heat prostration were CF sufferers. This led Di'Santagnese to the discovery of the greatly increased levels of salt in the sweat of people with CF. This has become the cornerstone on which the diagnosis of CF rests. A mother may notice a salty taste when she kisses her CF baby. Two physiologists, Gibson and Cooke, realized the need for a standard technique for collecting sweat for testing, and described a method of stimulating sweat production and collecting it.

One of the symptoms considered as an almost certain sign of CF was, in fact, first described in 1905 by Landsteiner. In translation, the title of his article reads: 'Intestinal obstruction from thickened meconium'. The first dark-green stools passed after birth are called meconium, and meconium ileus (an obstruction of the small intestine) affects 10–15 per cent of those infants destined to show the other signs of CF.

Poor absorption of food is a characteristic of most people with CF who go untreated. It manifests itself as steatorrhoea (non-digestion of fat leading to bulky, strong-smelling stools). There are also a number of other ways in which the disease may show its presence. In infants, the steatorrhoea may be accompanied by prolapse of the rectum (a condition where the very frequent passage of bulky stools causes the lining of the rectum to protrude through the anus). The first symptoms of CF in the young child are often confused with milk allergy.

Cystic fibrosis sufferers are also subject to recurrent chest infections. These are caused by bacteria, notably *Staphylococcus aureus* and the different types of *Pseudomonas*. While the former is an aggressive bacterium that causes disease in healthy people, the latter is an opportunist, that requires a weakness in the tissue it is attacking before it can gain a foothold. Conditions in the lungs of CF patients provide the right environment for both organisms to thrive and generally, although not always, one or other organism is found. Before anti-staphyloccal antibiotics were discovered, *Staphylococcus aureus* predominated. The effects of

11

repeated chest infections usually led to death by seven years of age. Now, survival is much longer and a progression from staphylococcal to pseudomonal infection is common in those patients more severely affected.

As suggested above, there is great variation in the severity of CF, even within members of the same family. A number of studies have shown that girls with CF generally do slightly worse than boys. Nevertheless, a good number of affected girls have grown up to have children. The vast majority of men with CF are sterile; Shwachman showed in 1968 that this was due to fibrosis of the epididymus and vas deferens (the organ and duct through which sperm pass on their way from the testis to the exterior of the body; see Figure 7).

Puberty may be delayed in CF sufferers, especially if they are underweight and undersized for their age. These symptoms can result in psychological problems in adolescence. The child may question treatment at this stage and normal adolescent rebellion can result in the breaking of dietary restrictions and resistance to physiotherapy and taking medicines.

Cystic fibrosis is a hereditary disease. Cedric Carter, in 1952, was the first to recognize the way in which the CF gene is transmitted from one generation to the next. The disease is caused by a pair of abnormal *recessive* genes in each cell of the body (a gene is a small portion of the genetic material, that is concerned with the making of a protein). The effects of a single recessive gene are masked when the normal form of the same gene also occurs in the same cell in a carrier. The defective gene in CF is on an autosome; occurring equally often in males and females (this is discussed further in Chapter 4). The illness CF affects only those individuals who have inherited the defective gene from *both* their mother and father. If two carriers marry there is a one in four chance that any of their offspring may inherit the gene from each of them. No adverse health problems occur for the parents through being carriers.

What is cystic fibrosis

It has become clear that CF is the commonest autosomal recessive genetic disease of white Indo-Europeans (Caucasians). In most parts of the world, between 1 in 1500 and 1 in 2500 Caucasian children are born with CF, though the disease may not be apparent at birth. If one takes these two sets of figures and assumes that all CF arises from the same genetic defect, then between 1 in 16 and 1 in 25 Caucasians is a carrier. No reliable test to detect a CF carrier exists. We only know of carrier status after the birth of a CF child to a particular couple. However, very recent research advances may allow detection of carriers in some families where CF has already occurred.

On average, one child with CF is born every day in the United Kingdom, and four to five daily in the United States. In fact, the condition occurs wherever Europeans have settled. It is extremely rare in the Chinese, and in the Negro races in Africa. In some Third World countries, with high infant mortality, a diagnosis of CF could easily be missed. In Britain, we occasionally see CF in children of Pakistani and Arab descent. The incidence in their countries of origin is unknown.

The precise nature of the CF gene itself is still unclear, although it has recently been found to be located on chromosome 7, linked to other known genes. Major research work on chromosome 7 could perhaps tell us more about the gene in the not too distant future.

Despite the lack of information on the basic defect, an aggressive approach to treatment has resulted in increased survival and health for CF sufferers. Time out of school or off work has been reduced through better attention to chest infections, a positive attitude to chest physiotherapy, attention to the special diet, and early recognition of danger signs. Treatment is best co-ordinated in a multidisciplinary CF clinic and is mostly on an out-patient basis. Certain treatments have not stood the test of time. Notable among these is the use of mist tents, in which affected children used to sleep (careful study showed these to be of no value in lessening the effects of the disease). We continue to search for effective treatments and to question the necessity of treatments that involve sacrifice of time or convenience by the affected person. Unfortunately, many of the effective treatments do require such sacrifice.

There is controversy about many aspects of CF: the basic causes of the disease, its evolution, changes that occur as it progresses, and its treatment. To write a book about 'the facts' is not easy and our own intuition and prejudice about various theories will be evident. However, we have tried hard to be objective and to highlight the more readily accepted points.

2

What is happening in the body in cystic fibrosis?

Three main systems in the body are classically affected by cystic fibrosis. These are the lungs and respiratory tract, the digestive system (particularly the pancreas and intestines) and the sweat glands. In this chapter the effects of CF on each of these three systems will be discussed in more detail.

THE LUNGS AND RESPIRATORY TRACT

Figure 1 shows the normal anatomy of the respiratory tree. Air enters through the nostrils into the nasal sinuses, then passes into the single tube of the trachea or windpipe. The trachea splits at its bottom end into two bronchi (one for each lung), and the bronchi continue to divide into smaller and smaller tubes (bronchioles), ending in thousands of small air sacs or alveoli. It is from the alveoli that oxygen enters the bloodstream and carbon dioxide is released.

From the upper airways down to the bronchioles, the respiratory tree is lined with many small, hair-like protrusions called cilia. The cilia are covered in a thin layer of mucus. They beat in a wave-like motion to waft the mucus and any extraneous matter (including bacteria) towards the nose or pharynx. Whatever reaches the upper part of the respiratory tree is either swallowed or coughed out. Ciliary action will normally act against gravity to clear the various lobes of the lung, whatever position the body may be in.

In CF however, mucus tends to clog up the upper and lower respiratory tree. The reasons for this are not clear. Though it would be attractive to ascribe this to abnormally

15

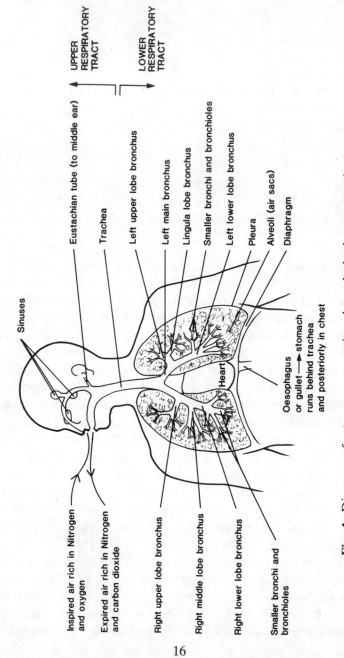

Fig. 1. Diagram of a transverse section through the human respiratory tree.

What is happening in the body in cystic fibrosis?

low water content of the mucus or to uneven ciliary beating, detailed research has not proved that either of these mechanisms is responsible. However, there is no doubt that mucus is poorly cleared against gravity in the presence of bacterial infection.

Build-up of mucus in the lungs can have several consequences. Ball-valve effects occur in those segments of the lung that have become overdistended because air passes an obstruction on breathing in, but does not all pass back on breathing out. These obstructions are caused by mucus and airway narrowing. The overinflation becomes more marked with time, and results in emphysema, a state of overdistension in which the elasticity of the lung is reduced. Deformity of the chest develops, with rounding of the shoulders and prominence of the sternum. Occasionally, and usually late in the course of the disease, distended alveoli at the surface of the lung may rupture, giving rise to pneumothorax (air between the surface of the lung and the chest wall) requiring special treatment. This damage is compounded by recurrent or continuous chest infections, or by bronchiectasis, a state of permanent weakening of the bronchial walls and poor drainage of infected mucus. Bronchiectasis is associated with permanent lung infection and clubbing of the fingers (see Fig. 2). Clubbing occurs as a result of substances associated

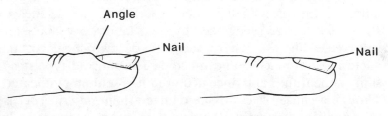

Fig. 2. Diagram of finger clubbing (see also Key to Fig. 9).

17

with the lung infections entering the blood. In some way these stimulate the growth of the soft tissue at the bases of the finger and toenails, causing loss of the angle between the nail and the skin. Abnormalities in the air and blood supply to the lungs may result from CF. These abnormalities may not be immediately apparent, as the reserve capacity of the lungs allows them to function normally even when quite significantly damaged. Studies with radioactive compounds either injected into a vein or inhaled (see Chapter 3, p. 43, and Fig. 10) can show the extent of the tissue damage.

Bacterial infections in the respiratory tree in CF

Though a number of bacterial chest infections may occur in CF, the commonest is caused by *Staphylococcus aureus*. Later in the course of the disease, infection by *Pseudomonas* bacteria may also occur. *Staphylococcus aureus* is a microorganism that does not occur in the body naturally, but only as part of an infection. It may cause minor problems such as pimples, or more major ones like osteomyelitis (a bone infection) in the general population, but in CF it is found together with chronic (long-term) bronchitis and lung infection. The bacterium *Pseudomonas aeruginosa* does not infect healthy tissue. It only attacks damaged tissue, for example the skin in severe burns, or the lungs in CF, when a certain degree of damage and loss of some of the healthy lining of the bronchi has occurred. Different varieties of *Pseudomonas* are recognized by their laboratory characteristics (see Fig. 3). There seem to be two forms of the bacteria, non-mucoid and mucoid. The mucoid type has a slimy appearance and once acquired it is seldom eradicated. Though a cause of less tissue damage than *Staphylococcus*, an established mucoid *Pseudomonas* infection is generally associated with deterioration in lung function.

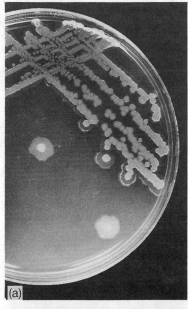

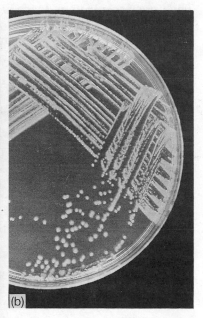

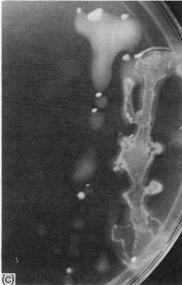

Fig. 3. Photographs of non-mucoid and mucoid *Pseudomonas* colonies on Agar culture plates. (a) non-mucoid – rough; (b) non-mucoid – smooth; (c) mucoid.

The upper respiratory tract in CF

Cystic fibrosis may cause changes in the nose and in other parts of the respiratory tree above the trachea. Nasal polyps (protruberant growths of the mucous membranes) develop in the nose in many older children. They occasionally require surgical removal, but have a tendency to recur.

THE GASTRO-INTESTINAL TRACT

The effects of CF on the gastro-intestinal tract are numerous and complex. To help understand them more fully, an outline of the normal processes of digestion and metabolism of food is given below.

Introduction to digestion and metabolism

In the normal digestive process, food is broken down both mechanically (chewing) and chemically from complex molecules such as proteins, fats, and carbohydrates (starch) to smaller, simpler molecules such as amino acids, fatty acids and sugars. This allows the food to be absorbed into the body through the walls of the small intestine or ileum (see Fig. 4), and then transported in the blood to the liver. The liver is the central chemical factory of the body: here the amino acids and other small molecules are used as building blocks for the body's own proteins, carbohydrates, etc. These then circulate in the bloodstream and are taken up by the various body tissues (e.g. lungs, muscles, brain etc.) as they need them. Tissues need a constant supply of proteins and other nutrients because many cells live only a few days or weeks and there is a constant replacement of dead or dying cells.

Let us look briefly at the individual food types and their fates.

What is happening in the body in cystic fibrosis?

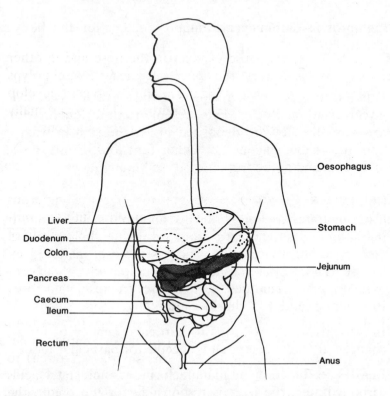

Fig. 4. Diagram of a transverse section through the human digestive system.

Proteins

Proteins are made of long chains of amino acids, coiled into complex shapes. In the digestive system they are broken down first into peptides (short amino acid chains), then to individual amino acids. Proteins serve many functions in the body. They are essential for tissue growth and repair, and enzymes (the molecules that speed up and control the many thousands of chemical reactions in the body) are proteins. In long-term infections or diseases like CF, large amounts of protein are needed for constant tissue repair, and even a high-protein diet may not supply enough for the body's needs.

Fats

Fats and oils are broken down in the digestive system to glycerol and fatty acids. Fats are important for energy storage: for this they are deposited under the skin in what is known as subcutaneous fat. Other functions of fats are as lubricants and in the formation of cell membranes.

Carbohydrates (starch)

Carbohydrates are long, branched and unbranched chains of polysaccharides. They are broken down to shorter chains, and thence to disaccharides such as sucrose, maltose, and lactose. These disaccharides are then split into their component monosaccharides (e.g. glucose, fructose, galactose). Both mono- and disaccharides are referred to as sugars.

In the tissues, proteins in particular undergo further changes, to make compounds specific for particular tissues.

Besides its function in manufacturing proteins, fats, and carbohydrates, the liver is responsible for the breakdown and detoxification of waste products in the body. These waste products then pass out of the body in the urine or faeces. The body uses only glucose products in metabolism and so, in the liver, all monosaccharides are converted to glucose compounds. Glucose is the main fuel for the chemical cycle that supplies energy for the body's functions. Ready glucose energy is stored in the liver and muscles as glycogen. When glycogen stores are full, the excess is stored as fat.

The digestive tract

The parts of the digestive tract (see Fig. 4) involved in each step of digestion are as follows. In the mouth food particles are reduced in size by the teeth and the digestion of starch begins with the action of the enzyme amylase present in saliva. The smell and taste of food stimulate the production of saliva and also of gastrin, a hormone which acts on the stomach to stimulate the production of enzymes there. After being swallowed, food travels down the oesophagus or gullet to the stomach. (Transport of food through the digestive tract is achieved by the action of muscles in the gut wall). Food stays in the stomach for about four hours, during which time it mixes with hydrochloric acid and the enzyme pepsin (pepsin is responsible for breaking down the protein in the diet to peptides). The food is prevented from leaving the stomach by a valve called the pylorus, which closes off the entrance to the duodenum. The presence of food in the stomach stimulates the production of a hormone (see Glossary for definition) called secretin. This hormone travels in the bloodstream to the duodenum, the liver, and the pancreas, where it stimulates the production of digestive juices.

After four hours in the stomach the food is in the form of a ball or bolus. The pyloric valve then opens, and this bolus of food passes into the duodenum. There it encounters an alkaline digestive fluid consisting of bicarbonate, bile, and the enzymes trypsin, amylase, and lipase from the pancreas. Trypsin completes the breaking down of peptides to amino acids. Amylase continues with the breaking down of starch to the disaccharides sucrose, maltose, and lactose. Further enzymes from the walls of the duodenum itself break down the disaccharides to their component monosaccharides. Fats are emulsified by the bile and then broken down by lipase to glycerol and fatty acids.

From the duodenum, the food travels slowly down through the jejunum and ileum. This whole section of the digestive tract is lined with tiny villi, folds in the gut lining, that increase the surface area available for food absorption. Amino acids, monosaccharides, and the smaller fat breakdown products are absorbed into the blood vessels lining the villi and transported from there to the liver. Larger fat breakdown products enter the lymph channels or lacteals. (The lymphatic system, like the blood system, transports materials around the body and helps to defend it from infection.) In the lymph channels the fat particles are coated, rendering them more soluble, before they enter the bloodstream and eventually reach the liver.

Certain substances in the diet that cannot be digested act as roughage, helping to increase the bulk of the bolus and help its passage down the intestinal canal. Notable amongst these is a polysaccharide, raffinose, which forms the fibres in many vegetables. The process of digestion continues all the way down to the end of the ileum.

At the end of the ileum, undigested material passes into the caecum, a mixing chamber. From there it enters the colon where much of the water is reabsorbed. Bacteria normally present in the caecum and colon act on the waste products to break them down into faeces by a process of fermentation. The fermentation also results in the formation of gas (flatus or wind). If there is poor absorption of food, especially of fat, this process of fermentation is especially active, and faeces and flatus become foul-smelling. This happens in a person with CF either taking a diet too rich in fat or receiving too little pancreatic supplement. Carbohydrates can also ferment in the intestine, though special forms of carbohydrate such as Caloreen® and Maxijoule® are less subject to fermentation. These compounds can be used in CF to increase energy intake without unpleasant side-effects.

The pancreas and CF

As has already been mentioned, one of the major effects of cystic fibrosis is on the pancreas. Replacement of pancreatic cells with fibrous scar tissue begins before birth, and generally gets worse with time. As a result of this tissue damage, caused initially by deposits of dried up secretions, the pancreas ceases to function properly. Production of pancreatic juices decreases, and as we saw previously this juice contains enzymes essential for the breakdown and absorption of food. In this section we will look in more detail at the function of the pancreas and how it is affected by CF.

The pancreas secretes mainly water, bicarbonate, and protein enzymes. Secretion of pancreatic juices is a continuous process, but the presence of food in the stomach, or certain other stimuli, can increase the rate of secretion. Bicarbonate secreted in the pancreatic juice is essential in changing the pH of the duodenal contents from the acidic stomach pH to the alkaline pH at which pancreatic enzymes function best. (pH is a measure of acidity or alkalinity).

Pancreatic enzymes are responsible for the breakdown of many components of the diet. Brief descriptions of the actions of the three major pancreatic enzymes were given in the previous section. After absorption and entry into the bloodstream these building blocks provide the essential substances for body growth and repair and the fuels on which the body functions.

Malabsorption

As described earlier, when foodstuffs are not adequately digested they cannot be absorbed normally from the intestines. This results in a wide range of symptoms due to abnormal excretion of fat in the faeces (steatorrhoea) and deficiency of vitamins soluble in fat, as well as proteins, minerals, carbohydrates, other vitamins, and water. Steatorrhoea is a major problem in inadequately treated CF. Furthermore, because the fat is only partly digested, it causes irritation of the bowel and this in turn leads to an increase in the frequency and rate of passage of bowel contents.

Deficiency of the enzyme trypsin means that some of the

protein in the diet is not fully broken down to amino acids in the duodenum. Some peptide fragments remain, and since these cannot be absorbed, they pass into the lower intestine and bowel. Here they are broken down to amino acids by other enzymes and by bacteria. As a result, large amounts of amino acids find their way into the faeces, where together with undigested fat they produce a pronounced odour.

The obvious treatment for malabsorption of food is to try and supplement the levels of natural digestive enzymes. Simultaneously, factors that are lacking from the diet due to abnormal digestion and absorption must be introduced into the body by some other route in order to prevent malnutrition. These therapeutic approaches are dealt with in more detail in Chapter 3. Since pancreatic enzymes do not reach the intestine in CF, pancreatic enzyme supplements are an essential part of treatment.

Gastro-intestinal symptoms of CF

During the newborn period: meconium ileus

The first stools of a newborn baby are called meconium. Ten to fifteen per cent of the babies with CF have intestinal obstruction in the first few days of life. The small intestine is clogged with sticky meconium, presumably because of thickened mucus from the intestinal glands. This blockage of the lower intestine causes bilious vomiting and swelling of the abdomen. X-rays help to distinguish meconium ileus from other causes of intestinal blockage.

Surgery is generally necessary in meconium ileus, though the administration of hygroscopic (water-attracting) enemas or the use of other substances capable of thinning mucus may occasionally be effective. The most successful operation has been Bishop and Koop's ileostomy. This entails bringing a loop of the ileum to open on the abdominal wall. Stools can then be passed above the blockage, while medication can be given through the opening to clear the obstruction (see Fig. 5). Once the lower bowel has been unblocked, stools can once again pass along the normal channel and the ileostomy can be closed. This generally takes between one and three months to happen. The immediate prognosis (i.e. chances of recovery from) of meconium ileus improved markedly after introduction of the ileostomy operation in the late 1960s.

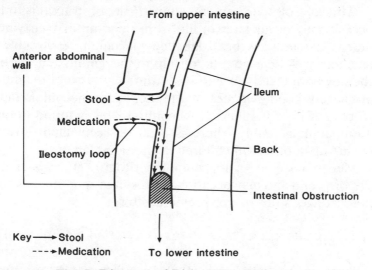

Fig. 5. Diagram of Bishop–Koop ileostomy.

Care of newborn babies before and after operations has improved greatly in the last ten years. As a result, it has become possible for some infants with meconium ileus to have a much simpler operation. In the new operation the most obstructed part of the bowel is simply removed, and the two cut ends are joined.

It is a myth to suppose that children born with meconium ileus and thus diagnosed as having CF at birth are less prone to lung disease. While meconium ileus almost always implies the presence of CF in Caucasians, this is not invariable. Confirmation of CF by the sweat test is very important in any case of meconium ileus.

The most serious complication of meconium ileus is meconium peritonitis, an acute inflammation of the membrane that lines the abdomen (the peritoneum). Meconium peritonitis may be present at birth. It occurs when a hole develops in the wall of a section of bowel blocked by meconium. The meconium spills into the peritoneum and causes inflammation.

Attacks of incomplete intestinal obstruction may occasionally occur later in life from build-up of faeces and mucus. These have been labelled meconium ileus equivalent, but they bear no relationship to the condition affecting the newborn (see later in this section).

There is good evidence of a tendency for meconium ileus to recur within families. If meconium ileus is found in one member of a family, there is a 50 per cent chance of it occurring in other CF children in the same family.

Meconium ileus or meconium peritonitis may affect the unborn child and may occasionally result in spontaneous late miscarriage, stillbirth, or premature birth.

After the newborn period

Symptoms of gastro-intestinal abnormalities in CF are often seen before symptoms in the respiratory system or elsewhere. The most pronounced symptom is steatorrhoea, fatty or loose, strong-smelling stools. It is often associated with abdominal distension. Steatorrhoea is the indirect result of the fibrous scarring of the pancreas from which CF derives its name. The fibrous tissue blocks the ducts of the pancreas and eventually stops the pancreatic digestive juices from reaching the small intestine to digest the food. This process, which is already well established by birth, in turn causes nutrients to be inefficiently absorbed. It is poor digestion of fat, particularly, that gives the faeces in steatorrhoea their characteristic look, hence the name steatorrhoea (*steato* being the Greek word for fat, and *rhoia* for flowing). Certain amino acids do not depend on the pancreas for breakdown but are nevertheless poorly absorbed, showing that the small intestine itself is not functioning perfectly in CF.

Rectal prolapse. In this condition, malabsorption of fat, with very frequent stools, results in the inner lining of the rectum protruding through the anus. CF should be considered in any infant with a prolapsed rectum. Rectal prolapse should come under ready control if dietary fat is reduced and pancreatic enzymes are given with the feeds.

Meconium ileus equivalent. This rather poor term is used for attacks of complete or partial intestinal obstruction that may occur later on in the life of a person with CF. Attacks occur mainly as a result of blockage caused by mucus and fatty stools. In some CF adults abdominal pain and attacks of such obstruction may be the main complaint. The condition is not more common amongst those who had meconium ileus at birth. Recent improvements in the treatment of CF have reduced the incidence of this complication.

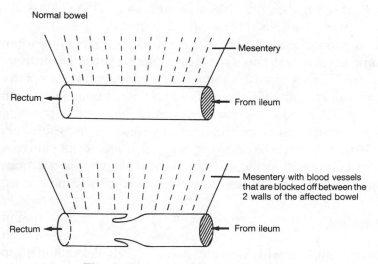

Fig. 6. Diagram of intussusception.

Intussusception. In this disorder a portion of small intestine closer to the stomach folds into the adjoining region of the downstream bowel, threatening the blood supply of the trapped inner portion (see Fig. 6). Intussusception is a rare but potentially serious complication of CF. Treatment is nearly always by operation.

The liver and biliary tree

Cirrhosis (fibrous scarring) of the liver occurs in about 5 per cent of people with CF. In this disorder, the fibrous tissue laid down partially blocks the veins draining into the liver from the intestine and spleen. As the fibrous tissue contracts (part of the natural progression of any fibrotic process), the liver cells may be damaged. As a result they are unable to carry out their normal tasks. The partial blockage of the blood supply to the spleen causes it to enlarge, and the veins at the lower end of the oesophagus may also become swollen and varicosed. These varices (or dilated veins) may bleed on occasion and require the injection of sclerosing agents, which strengthen the blood vessel wall. Though this is a potentially serious complication that can cause jaundice, liver failure, and bleeding, in CF it is more common to see mild cases, which run a course over many years. Even after a more serious manifestation, the condition may improve. Why only a few CF patients have this complication is not fully understood. It is not necessarily the older or the more severely ill who are affected in this way. The newborn with CF may sometimes show prolonged jaundice, possibly because of mucus in the bile channels. This resolves with time and is not especially associated with liver disease later in life.

Diabetes

Most children with diabetes have so-called insulin-dependent diabetes. Two hormones, insulin and glucagon, are produced by the pancreas, in groups of cells known as the Islets of Langerhans. Glucagon is produced by alpha cells in these regions, while insulin is produced by beta cells. Insulin lowers the levels of sugar (glucose) in the blood by converting it to the carbohydrate glycogen, which is stored in the liver. Glucagon is one of the hormones that reconverts glycogen to glucose.

In insulin-dependent diabetes most of the beta cells (those manufacturing insulin) are destroyed. However, diabetes in people with CF is caused by contraction of fibrous scar tissue, which destroys limited numbers of both alpha and beta cells. The resulting diabetes, which may first appear in the early teens, is generally mild and easily controlled with small doses of insulin. The more severe complications of diabetes such as coma and acidosis (a build up of acids in the blood) are unusual. Long-term kidney complications do not occur. About 3 per cent of adolescents and adults with CF develop diabetes.

Rare gastro-intestinal manifestations in CF

Oedema is a generalized body swelling caused by low levels of the protein albumin in the blood. Albumin is involved in the process of keeping fluid in the blood vessels. When albumin is deficient, fluid builds up in the tissues. Oedema is sometimes found as a sign of cystic fibrosis in young infants. On occasion this has happened when the first loose stools have been misdiagnosed as milk allergy and soya feeds have been given.

Absence of gastro-intestinal symptoms

A small proportion of people with CF have no problems with their digestive system. This lack of symptoms is difficult to understand. Some studies claim that as many as 10 per cent of CF patients show no gastro-intestinal problems. The diagnosis of CF may be suspect in some of this 10 per cent. On the other hand, if one only suspects CF when there *are* gastro-intestinal symptoms, one may underdiagnose this category of patients.

THE SWEAT GLAND

Sweat consists of a weak solution of electrolytes (electrically charged molecules) in water. These are mainly sodium and chloride, with some calcium and some potassium. The electrolyte solution has the same pH as the blood, being slightly alkaline. In CF there is a marked increase of these electrolytes in the sweat, because the reabsorption of chloride is impaired. The reason for this impaired absorption has not yet been established. Unlike other organs affected by CF, the sweat gland and its duct appear normal when examined under the microscope.

THE REPRODUCTIVE SYSTEM

One of the most consistent findings in men with CF is an abnormality of the epididymus and vas deferens (the tubes that carry sperm from the testes (see Fig. 7). These tubes end in blind channels instead of connecting through to the urethra. At least 97 per cent of males with CF are affected in this way from birth. As a result, most men with CF are sterile, although there have been documented cases of men with CF producing normal sperm and, in a few instances, of fathering children.

There are no equivalent changes in the female reproductive tract, and more than 100 women with CF have been reported as giving birth to children. In two reported instances the children born also had CF. (Of course, all children born to a woman with CF must of necessity be carriers of the disease; see Chapter 4.) Occasionally, reduced amounts of the mucus that normally lubricates the

What is happening in the body in cystic fibrosis?

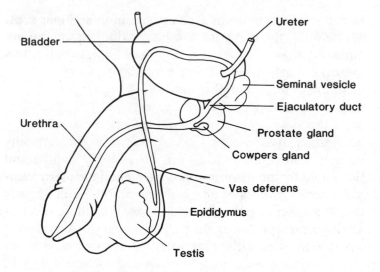

Fig. 7. Diagram of the male reproductive system.

female reproductive tract causes infertility in women with CF.

A BRIEF SUMMARY OF HOW CF MAY ANNOUNCE ITSELF

In the newborn:
intestinal obstruction caused by meconium ileus or atresia;
prolonged jaundice.
Infants:
rectal prolapse;
recurrent loose stools;
distended abdomen;
'milk allergy';
recurrent chestiness, coughing or wheezing;
a salty taste to the sweat;
poor weight gain, often associated with a ravenous appetite;
unexplained dehydration.

Because such symptoms are very common and may sometimes be mild, the diagnosis can be overlooked in infancy.
In older children:
    after the diagnosis of CF in a brother or sister;
    incomplete intestinal obstruction;
    nasal polyps, especially if recurrent;
    bronchiectasis or recurrent chest infections;
    heat prostration;
    underweight child.
    Occasionally the diagnosis may be missed for many years.
In adolescents or adults:
    delayed onset of puberty;
    sterile or azospermic males;
    infertile females with scanty cervical mucus.

HOW IS A DIAGNOSIS OF CF CONFIRMED?

In most circumstances, CF can be confirmed in children by a carefully performed sweat test. In the sweat test, a small amount of pilocarpine (a sweating promoter) is driven into the skin by stimulation with a few amperes of electric current (this process is known as iontophoresis). When the sweating rate is adequate, the concentrations of sodium and chloride (i.e. salt) in the sweat are measured.

In a normal child the sweat will contain sodium and chloride in concentrations of between fifteen and thirty millimoles per litre (mmol l^{-1}). Concentrations of sodium and chloride greater than 70 mmol l^{-1} are diagnostic of CF. This means that children with CF have two to five times the normal amount of salt in their sweat. A concentration of sodium and choride well above 70 mmol l^{-1} does not indicate that the disease will be more severe.

The sweat test is quite safe and very reliable, but it needs to be performed by experienced staff. Stimulation of an adequate sweating rate in very young infants can sometimes be a problem. The recent introduction of a system that employs capillary pressure to suck up sweat into polythene tubing has made sweat testing easier and more efficient, though the equipment used is very expensive.

The sweat test is the least unpleasant method of diagnosis. In cases where the results of this test are borderline, it may be necessary to measure the pancreatic secretions directly, and check whether these secretions are reaching the duodenum. For this test it used to be necessary to insert a small tube into the duodenum via the mouth, but the test can now be done more simply by taking a urine sample and measuring substances in the urine that depend on pancreatic function.

It should be noted that in people with CF who have no intestinal troubles (see earlier section), the pancreatic secretion results would be near normal.

Occasionally, CF may go undiagnosed for many years, in which case it could be necessary to recognize the disease in an adult. For adults, the normal range of salt concentration in sweat is greater than for children, and the sweat test rather loses its value in diagnosis. Men thought to have CF can be tested for azospermia (absence of sperm in the ejaculate).

SHOULD WE SCREEN THE NEWBORN FOR CF?

The validity of testing all newborn babies for CF is still a matter of debate. A simple test (BM Meconium) exists, which works on the principle that the albumin content of the meconium is increased in newborns with CF. This has been used in some countries over the past decade. A more reliable test is the measurement of serum immune-reactive trypsin (IRT) in a specimen of blood. This test is based on the observed reaction of the body's antibody defences to the pancreatic enzyme trypsin. A raised level of the antibody is found in the blood of most newborns with CF.

Advantages and problems of screening

One argument in favour of screening all newborn children for CF is that if the very early changes caused by the disease can be identified, they may throw new light on the way that the disease progresses. Studies on both the tests mentioned above have already proved useful.

There are, however, problems with both the screening tests available at present. Neither of the current tests give a conclusive diagnosis — for a screening test to identify a high percentage of children with CF, the sensitivity needs to be set very high. This inevitably results in some babies who do not have CF getting positive tests. In one study in East Anglia using the IRT test, of 20 036 consecutive births screened, there were 0.28 per cent false positives, i.e. 56 babies who did not have CF gave a positive test result. These babies presumably had temporary high trypsin levels and needed a second blood test before CF could be excluded. Knowledge that a child had a positive screening test would be unpleasant for the parents, even more so if later tests showed the first one to be false. Great care is needed in the conveying of the results of abnormal screening tests. Nine of the 20 000 babies in the East Anglian study had persistently high IRT levels and of these eight proved to have CF. The cause of the raised level in the ninth child, who was still well at 14 months, was uncertain. One ethical problem which needed attention during the development of this screening programme was whether to inform parents of positive results or simply to tell their medical practitioners and wait until the onset of symptoms to do a sweat test.

There are also occasional false *negatives* in the IRT screening test, though with the varying age of onset and of diagnosis in CF, the true error rate is difficult to determine. One convenient aspect of the IRT test is that the amount of blood needed is very small. The test can be easily performed on the same specimen of blood that is routinely collected at

about 10 days of age from every newborn baby, for phenyl-
ketonuria (another hereditary disease) and thyroid function
screening.

The most controversial question relating to newborn
screening for CF is whether the eventual prognosis is altered
by early diagnosis. This remains extraordinarily difficult to
prove. Unfortunately, the strongest argument for screening
remains the ease with which a diagnosis of CF may be
overlooked, some children having had symptoms for a long
time before the diagnosis of CF is considered or made. In
one study, the *average* delay between onset of symptoms
(excluding meconium ileus) and diagnosis was 13 months.
This delay can cause psychological problems — parents may
feel guilty about not noticing ill effects earlier, or may blame
the general practitioner for not recognizing the symptoms
when he first saw the child.

By allowing very early diagnosis, screening would sometimes prevent the birth of a second affected child.

If a truly effective early treatment for CF becomes available, capable of greatly reducing damage to the pancreas
and lungs, then the case for screening would be made. Until
then, screening will continue to depend on the enthusiasm of
practitioners and laboratory directors in certain regions. In
areas with no screening test, it is important that paediatricians educate themselves, general practitioners, and the
public about the early signs of CF.

3

Treatment of cystic fibrosis

THE CF CLINIC — A MULTIDISCIPLINARY APPROACH

Treatment of CF in a special clinic allows a local body of expertise to build up, to help manage the many complex ways in which the illness can affect a person. Greater longevity and improved health have been directly ascribed to special clinic treatment as opposed to care of the child by the paediatrician or medical practitioner alone.

An efficient CF clinic has a team of trained staff. The team is led by a paediatrician and consists of a nursing sister, who works exclusively with CF patients (she has home and hospital contact with the families); a physiotherapist interested in sports medicine and lung function; a dietician; a psychologist; and a social worker. The parents are the most important members of the treatment team, and later the child him/herself. Continuity is the greatest secret of success. At the clinic at the Royal Manchester Children's Hospital (RMCH), the nursing assistant who helps at the clinic has been attached to it for 10 years and knows all sorts of family details which have proved important from time to time. We believe patients can be better treated at a special CF clinic than at a respiratory or gastro-intestinal clinic that includes patients with CF. Unless there are insuperable geographical problems, a CF clinic should probably have a minimum of 10 patients and a maximum of 40 to each paediatrician. A recent working party of the British Paediatric Association recommended that each affected person should be known to a major CF clinic, with care shared between this clinic, paediatricians, physicians, and local general practitioners.

Treatment of cystic fibrosis

With improved survival, more 'adult' CF clinics are coming into being. The age at which patients move to thc adult clinic varies according to local facilities and expertise, but it may be as early as 16 years old. In some centres the physician and paediatrician run joint clinics and achieve continuity that way.

At the RMCH the 60 patients we have at present attend the weekly clinic by appointment where possible, though at any other time an open door policy operates to clinic attendance and to the in-patients ward. The patient and parents will see the paediatrician on each visit to the clinic, and often see other members of the team informally in the large anteroom containing the scales and lung-function equipment. Team members might check on aspects of dietary care, or

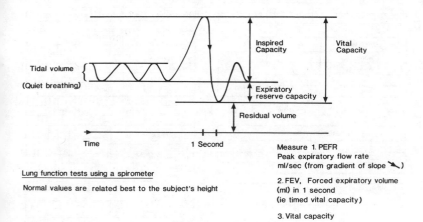

Measure 1. PEFR
Peak expiratory flow rate
ml/sec (from gradient of slope)

Lung function tests using a spirometer
Normal values are related best to the subject's height

2. FEV, Forced expiratory volume
(ml) in 1 second
(ie timed vital capacity)

3. Vital capacity

Fig. 8. Diagram to show the theory of lung function tests:
Key
Vital capacity = total volume of air that can be moved.
Inspired capacity = volume of air taken into the lungs on breathing in.
Expiratory reserve capacity = the extra volume of air which can be breathed out at the end of quiet expiration.
Residual volume = the air which remains in the lung after deepest expiration.

Cystic Fibrosis: the facts

ROYAL MANCHESTER CHILDREN'S HOSPITAL   CYSTIC FIBROSIS CLINIC

Name..   Date..............................Age...........Yrs. ....Mths.

Age decimal....................

GENERAL COMMENTS OR PROBLEMS

EXERCISE INTOLERANCE/HANDICAP	
None.	
Slight.	Joins in, but less endurance
Fair.	Rarely joins in, rapidly tires
Severe.	Immediate dyspnoea, often at rest

SCHOOL			
Normal		DAYS LOST	
Special			
Home Tutor		DAYS IN HOSPITAL	
Playschool			

COUGH	Day	Night
None		
After Pty		
Occasional		
Regular		
Frequent		

WHEEZE	
None	
Occasional	
Regular	

Haemoptysis   NO/YES   No.=

SPUTUM	Volume	
None		
After Pty		Clear
Little		Yellow
A lot		Green

PHYSIOTHERAPY	
Frequency	
F. E. Technique	Yes/No.
Percussor	Yes/No.
Aerosol	Yes/No
Self/Parent/Both	

NOSE   Obstruction ☐   Polyp ☐   Discharge/Runny ☐   Epistaxis ☐   Hayfever ☐

MEDICATION	
Antibiotic (oral)	
Bronchodilator	
DSCG	
Beclomethasone	
Nebulised antibiotic	
Other	

SUPPLEMENTS	Per Meal	Per Snack
Pancrex		
Pancrex V		
Cotazyme		
Nutrizyme		
Pancrease		
Cotazyme B		
Calories (Maxijoule, etc.)		
Protein (Vivonex, etc.)		
MCT		

LOW FAT DIET	Strict/Relaxed/Free Diet
APPETITE	Normal/Large/Reduced

STOOLS		
Average daily frequency		
Normal, formed		
Occasionally abnormal		Bulky
Frequently abnormal		Loose Smelly

BABY MILK	Type Quantity
WEANING DIET	

Fig. 9. A CF clinic recording chart or proforma. (From The Royal Manchester Children's Hospital Cystic Fibrosis Clinic.)

Treatment of cystic fibrosis

EXAMINATION   Height..........................(Cms.)   Weight.............................(Kgs.)

Pulse...............................   Respiratory rate.......................

CHEST SHAPE	Absent	Present	Severe
Sternal prominence			
Kyphosis			
Troughing			
Recession			

CLUBBING	
None	
Nail-bed hypertrophy	
"Watchglass" nails	
Drumsticks	

AUSCULTATION	Zone
Breath sounds	
Crackles	
Rhonchi	
Wheeze	

EARS

NOSE

SEXUAL MATURITY	I	II	III	IV
Pubic hair				
Breasts				
Penis				
Testicles				

THROAT

ABDOMEN

INVESTIGATIONS

CHANGES IN MANAGEMENT

COMMENTS

NEXT VISIT...

Key   Pty=physiotherapy
Dyspnoea=shortness of breath
Haemoptysis=the coughing of blood in sputum.
F.E. technique=forced-expiration technique, (huffing).
Epistaxis=bleeding from the nose.
DSCG=chromoglycate.
Clubbing:

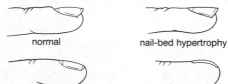

normal   nail-bed hypertrophy

watchglass   drumstick

Kyphosis=round-shouldered stooping.
Troughing=sucking in of lower chest with breathing in.
Recession=sucking in between the ribs with breathing in.
Ausculation=listening to chest through a stethoscope.

the efficiency of the parents' physiotherapy techniques in this way. Of course if a specific problem arises requiring detailed involvement of one of the team members (for example the psychologist), special arrangements can be made.

On a normal visit to the clinic, a patient is weighed, their height is recorded, and various measurements of lung function are taken. An instrument called a spirometer is used to measure lung function. The patient breathes into this apparatus, which measures the air capacity of the lungs, plus the speed and volume of air moved in and out of the lungs in breathing (see Fig. 8).

The findings of the physical examination are recorded on a proforma (Fig. 9), along with information on the patient's lung and bowel condition, their school or work attendance, and their treatment. The proforma shown in Fig. 9 is the one used at RMCH. We are encouraging neighbouring clinics in our region to use the same proforma so that computer comparisons can be made between subjects at different clinics.

After each clinic session, a round-table discussion of those people seen at the clinic or in the ward takes place between all the staff members. Aspects of management and any planned or on-going research are discussed in practical terms at this meeting. Patients are seen a minimum of once every three months at the RMCH clinic, but many have more frequent contact through home visits from the CF Nursing Sister.

The CF clinic: advantages and disadvantages

Advantages of a special CF clinic include improved health and life expectancy. A body of expert knowledge builds up and engenders confidence that the clinic is up to date with the latest advances in treatment. A cameraderie builds up between the children, their families and staff members, and there are improved research opportunities. Contact with subjects with more advanced disease and knowing affected people who die may be numbered among the disadvantages.

A question relating to CF clinics that is frequently asked is, 'Can one "catch" a *Pseudomonas* infection from someone else attending the clinic?' One very good study in Dublin has shown that only brothers and sisters tend to share the same *Pseudomonas* species. *Pseudomonas* is a very widespread micro-organism in nature, being found in any drainpipe, for instance. Person to person spread of the organism is likely to be of minor importance in CF.

Specific aspects of CF management

Chest X-ray films are taken at least once a year. These are scored according to an accepted system to allow formal comparison. In addition, a Shwachman score is estimated yearly. This score gives points on the basis of well-being, school attendance, chest symptoms and signs, growth and nutrition, and the X-ray results (see Table 1). Both scoring systems allow a more objective approach than is allowed by simply reacting to findings at any particular clinic visit. More recently, at RMCH we have been performing occasional chest scans on patients. These involve injecting and inhaling safe radioactive substances into the body. These penetrate the air and blood supply of the patient's lungs. Photographic scans of the chest may then show areas of the lungs receiving too little air or blood (see Fig. 10). Such areas may not be detectable by X-rays or with a stethoscope. Lung changes cannot always be detected with the stethoscope, and this makes the occasional performance of these other tests necessary.

The different tests of lung function are fairly variable and are more useful as indicators of long-term changes rather than being immediately useful.

Lung function tests can, however, have immediate use

Table 1. Clinical evaluation and grading criteria for patients with cystic fibrosis

Points	Case histories	Lungs, physical findings, and cough	Growth and nutrition	Chest X-ray
25	Full activity Normal exercise tolerance and endurance Normal strength Normal personality and disposition Normal school attendance	No cough Normal pulse and respiration No evidence of over-expansion Lungs clear to stethoscope Good posture No clubbing	Maintains weight and height well within normal range, or just like the rest of the family Good muscle development Normal amount of fat Normal sexual maturation Good appetite Well formed, almost normal stools	Normal
20	Slight limitation of strenuous activity Tires at end of day or after prolonged exertion Less energetic Low normal range of strength Occasionally irritable or lethargic Good school attendance	Occasional hacking cough Clearing of throat Resting pulse and respiration normal Mild over-expansion Occasional, usually localized, harsh breath sounds, wheezing or rattling mucus heard Good posture Mild clubbing	Maintains weight and height at slightly below average or the family normal Good muscle development Slighty decreased fat Slightly retarded sexual maturation Normal appetite Stools more frequent and slightly abnormal	Signs of excess air in slightly over-distended lungs

Treatment of cystic fibrosis

15	May rest voluntarily Tires after exertion Moderately inactive Slight weakness Lacking spontaneity Lethargic or irritable Fair school attendance	Mild chronic nonrepetitive cough in the morning on arising, after exertion or crying, or occasionally during the day No night cough Respiration and pulse *slightly* rapid Barrel chest Coarse breath sounds Occasional localized mucus rattling or wheezing Moderate rounding of shoulders Moderate clubbing	Maintains weight and height at lower end of normal and less than other family members Weight usually deficient for height Fair muscle development Moderately reduced fat Abdomen slightly distended Maturation definitely retarded Fair appetite Stools usually abnormal, large floating, occasionally foul, but formed	Excess air in over-distended lungs Distance from front to back of chest increased Diaphragm pushed down Blood vessels in lungs prominent Patches of lung with less air than normal
10	Limited physical activity and exercise tolerance Breathless after exertion Moderate weakness Fussy, irritable, sluggish or listless Poor school attendance, may require home tutor	Chronic cough, frequent, repetitive, productive and rarely paroxysmal Respiration and pulse moderately rapid Moderate to severe over-expansion Widespread sounds of wheezing and mucus rattling	Weight and height below normal Weight deficient for height Poor muscle strength Marked reduction in fat Abdomen distended Failure of sexual maturation and no adolescent growth spurt	As above, but more marked Heart shadow narrow from pressure of lungs

Table 1. Clinical evaluation and grading criteria for patients with cystic fibrosis

Points	Case histories	Lungs, physical findings, and cough	Growth and nutrition	Chest X-ray
10 (ctd)		Rounded shoulders and forward head Marked clubbing Usually blueness of tongue	Poor appetite Stools poorly formed, bulky, fatty and foul smelling	
5	Severe limitation of activity Breathless when standing or lying down Inactive or confined to bed or chair Marked weakness Apathetic or irritable Cannot attend school	Severe paroxysmal, frequent productive cough, often associated with vomiting or blood in sputum Night cough Rapid pulse or respiration Marked barrel chest Generalized squeaking, bubbly noises and wheezing heard Poor posture Severe clubbing	Malnourished and stunted Weak, flabby, small muscles Absence of fat Large, flabby, protruberant abdomen Failure to grow or gain weight, often with weight loss Bulky, frequent, foul, fatty stools Frequent rectal prolapse	Marked overdistension Cystic spaces between areas of lung receiving too little air

This system of clinical evaluation can be used to evaluate patients at each visit or at six- or twelve-month intervals in order to determine the severity of the disease and the effect of therapy in any one patient and to compare one patient with the next.

The physical findings and chest X-ray are the best indicators of the degree of lung involvement and may be used without the other indicators to simplify and shorten the scoring. After Shwachman H. and Kukzycki L. T. (1958) Long term study of 105 patients with cystic fibrosis: studies made over a 5–14-year period. *Am J Dis Child*, **96**, 6–15.

in detecting a bronchospasm (contraction of the bronchial tubes). Sometimes bronchospasm may be suspected but cannot be detected with a stethoscope. In these circumstances, lung function tests are carried out before and after administration of a bronchodilator, a substance that relaxes the bronchial tubes. If bronchospasm is present, then the bronchodilator will improve the condition, and this will show on the second lung function tests. A bronchodilator drug can then be prescribed to ease the bronchospasm.

Inoculation

Inoculation against those organisms that cause respiratory illness is advisable in CF. In particular, this applies to measles and pertussis (whooping cough), and unless there are very strong reasons not to, these inoculations should be performed. Most clinics immunize against influenza only if a potent strain is prevalent or forecast.

GENERAL ASPECTS OF CF TREATMENT

People with CF are encouraged to lead as normal and as active a life as possible. Children with CF who are swimming-fit, for instance, show improvement in their lung function and well-being. A cough is no bar to sporting activity, although, obviously, breathlessness does limit the activity of some. Experts in sports medicine are attached to some clinics.

Despite ignorance of the basic defect in CF, multidisciplinary treatment has greatly prolonged life and its quality, so that reaching adulthood in reasonable health is becoming the rule rather than the exception. However, the severity of symptoms in individuals is highly variable, and very severely affected children may still die of the disease despite excellent treatment. More disturbing are patients who are initially only mildly affected but enter a more serious category simply through neglect of treatment.

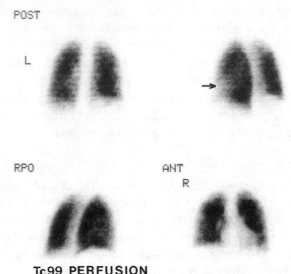

Tc99 PERFUSION

Fig. 10. A lung scan. Different panels show the lungs from different angles.

Perfusion tests are on the blood supply to various parts of the lung. Ventilation tests are on the distribution of inspired air to the various parts of the lung. Black areas on photographs are caused by radioactive emission. They denote lung tissue that is being well perfused or ventilated. White areas denote that the radioactive isotopes have not penetrated. Some of these areas are normal, and simply indicate the positions of the heart and spine. Other white areas denote parts of the lungs that are poorly perfused.

Though there are many contributing factors, the improved survival in CF has been largely due to the development of effective antibiotics against *Staphylococcus* bacteria and to more effective treatment of *Pseudomonas* infections. Flucloxacillin and the more expensive fucidic acid are the most common antibiotics used to prevent and treat staphylococcal

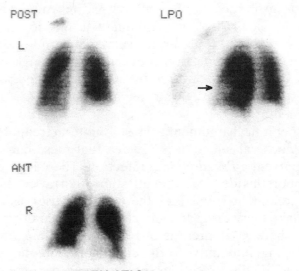

Kr81 VENTILATION

Fig. 10. (ctd) The two arrows in the figure mark an area of lung that is being poorly perfused and ventilated. This area was not obvious on listening to breathing with a stethoscope or on routine X-ray. Once found, special physiotherapy was applied to the particular zone.

Key: Tc99 = Technetium ⎫ radioactive isotopes that are inhaled (Tc99)
      Kr81 = Krypton ⎭ or given by injection (Kr81).
      L   = left   POST = posterior
      R   = right   LPO   = left posterior oblique
      ANT = anterior   RPO   = right posterior oblique

infections. There remain differences in practice between different clinics. Some, including ours at RMCH, believe in long-term (year-in, year-out) anti-staphylococcal treatment, using full therapeutic doses of either antibiotic mentioned above, given by mouth. We are able to eradicate the staphylococcal infection from the majority of our patients in this way. Other clinics prefer to treat a staphylococcal infection vigorously if it occurs. We believe that this can only be done safely in a CF clinic, with frequent testing for bacteria in sputum (phlegm) and careful surveillance. One danger of treating only the infection is that the family might not want to bother the doctor with a 'trivial' infection and some lung tissue damage may occur as a result of the delay in treatment.

A theoretical argument against long-term treatment of the staphylococcal infection is an idea that these bacteria may help prevent a *Pseudomonas* infection. There is no evidence to support this idea. Another question often raised about long-term treatment is whether the continual use of antibiotics can make these drugs less effective. Unlike many other bacteria, there is at present no evidence for *Staphylococcus* developing 'immunity' to the effects of antibiotics in CF.

Pseudomonas infections are difficult or impossible to eradicate. Once a mucoid *Pseudomonas* infection has become established it is generally a permanent feature, resulting in worsened lung function.

Current treatment can alleviate the infection by reducing the amount of sputum in the lungs and by keeping down the numbers of bacteria. Certain penicillins (e.g. azlocillin) together with aminoglycide drugs (e.g. netilmycin) are used to treat *Pseudomonas* infections. These drugs are given by injection into a vein. Other drugs that are sometimes used are the cephalosporins (e.g. ceftazidime), again given by injection. Courses of these drugs usually last about 10 days and are given in hospital where intensive physiotherapy and special attention to nutritional needs is possible. Sometimes these drugs or others (e.g. colimycin) that cannot be given by vein are given long-term by inhalation. One carefully controlled study of such inhalation in adults reported improved lung-function and well-being, with less days off work.

Difficulties of the treatment of pseudomonal infection are that most of the drugs used have to be given by injection, and may have unwelcome side-effects. That said, it is rare to see the usual adverse effects on hearing and kidney function from these drugs in CF. Some way of rendering the conditions in the lung less ideal for the *Pseudomonas* bacteria would seem the only way of eradicating pseudomonal infections. One approach has been to vaccinate against the bacteria, but this has proved ineffective. Another experiment that was attempted involved removing free calcium from the mucus in the lungs (*Pseudomonas* bacteria are known to thrive when free calcium is available). Unfortunately, this approach was also unsuccessful.

Cough suppressants or stimulants do not help CF patients with chest problems. This is because such compounds relieve symptoms but allow mucus to remain in the lungs, thus impairing their function.

In some patients with CF, there is bronchospasm with wheezing. This may be associated with the CF or may be due to the very common chest condition, asthma. Bronchospasm in CF patients is treated in the same way as asthma. Inhalation of the drug cromoglycate may be used to prevent bronchospasm. On occasion bronchodilators (e.g. salbutamol) and steroids that act on the lung surface (e.g. beclamethasone) may be given to some patients by inhalation.

Very occasionally, the airways may be washed out under anaesthetic (bronchial lavage) in an attempt to clear accumulated secretions preventing aeration of parts of the lung. In extreme cases a segment of lung with permanently dilated bronchi may be surgically removed. In some CF clinics in the USA and Canada such treatments are undertaken rather more often than in Great Britain.

PHYSIOTHERAPY IN CF

A fit person breathes more efficiently than an unfit one, especially when exercising. Someone with CF who is fit and has 'trained' their respiratory muscles is able to cope with the stresses of a chest infection more easily than an unfit person. The need for this 'training' may be especially marked in girls, since their muscles are often less well developed than those of boys. This is partly because of true sex differences in muscle bulk and strength, but differences are also partly cultural, with girls tending to play less active games inside, while boys are often more active outside. Girls with CF do slightly less well than boys at any age, and this may be partly because of weak chest muscles. This situation can be remedied by an active approach to physical exercise which develops the chest, especially swimming. People with CF who become swimming fit show an improvement in lung function.

It is precisely when the child is well that physiotherapy and chest muscle training are important. Some children and parents seem to think that paying attention to physiotherapy when the child has a cough is sufficient. Mucus in CF is relatively dehydrated, but if there is infection and the bronchi are dilated, secretions of mucus and sputum can be very copious. Clearance of these secretions is paramount in

---

Fig. 11. Positions for postural (bronchial) drainage. This series of illustrations shows the best positions for drainage of mucus from various parts of the lung. (All illustrations redrawn from Library of Congress Publication No. 74-21835, Cystic Fibrosis Foundation.)

(a) Diagram showing the various lobes of the lung.
(b) Postures for drainage of upper lobes of lung. (i) Apical segments; (ii) anterior segments; (iii) posterior segments.
(c) Drainage postures for lower lobes of lung. (i) Superior segments; (ii) anterior basal segments; (iii) lateral basal segments; (iv) posterior basal segments.
(d) Posture for drainage of lingular segments of left upper lobe.
(e) Drainage posture for right middle lobe of lung.
(f) Two positions in which the individual can perform self-therapy. (i) Upper lobe of lung, posterior segment. (ii) Right middle lobe of lung.

Treatment of cystic fibrosis

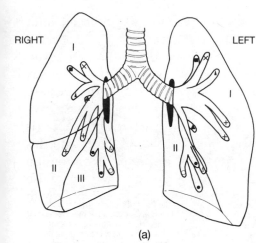

RIGHT   LEFT

Key:
I Upper lobe
× 1. Apical
▴ 2. Anterior
■ 3. Posterior
+ II 4–R Middle lobe – 4–L Lingula
  III Lower lobe
▲ 5. Superior
▵ 6. Anterior basal
• 7. Lateral basal
○ 8. Posterior basal

(a)

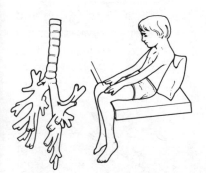

(i) Bed or drainage table flat. Patient leans back on pillow at 30° angle against therapist. Therapist claps with markedly cupped hand over area between clavicle (collarbone) and top of scapula (shoulder blade) on each side.)

(ii) Bed or drainage table flat . Patient lies back with pillow under knees. Therapist claps between clavicle (collarbone) and nipple on each side.

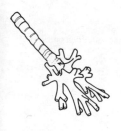

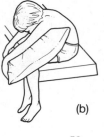

(iii) Bed or drainage table flat. Patient leans over folded pillow at 30° angle. Therapist stands behind and claps over upper back on both sides.

(b)

53

Cystic Fibrosis: the facts

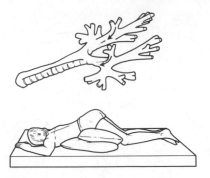

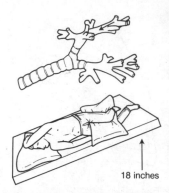

(i) Bed or table flat. Patient lies on abdomen with two pillows under hips. Therapist claps over middle of back at tip of scapula (shoulder blade), on either side of spine.

(ii) Foot of table or bed elevated 18 inches (about 30°). Patient lies on side, head down, pillow under knees. Therapist claps with slightly cupped hand over lower ribs. (Position shown is for drainage of *left* anterior basal segment. To drain the right anterior basal segment, patient should lie on his left side in same posture.)

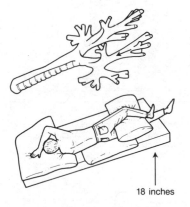

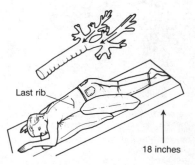

(iii) Foot of table or bed elevated 18 inches (about 30°). Patient lies on abdomen, head down, then rotates ¼ turn upward. Upper leg is flexed over pillow for support. Therapist claps over uppermost portion of lower ribs. (Position shown is for drainage of *right* lateral basal segment. To drain the left lateral basal segment, patient should lie on his right side in the same posture.)

(iv) Foot of table or bed elevated 18 inches (about 30°). Patient lies on abdomen, head down, with pillow under hip. Therapist claps over lower ribs close to spine on each side.

(c)

Treatment of cystic fibrosis

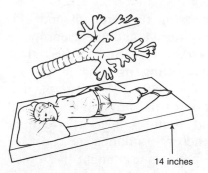

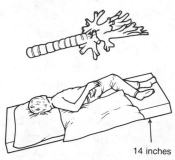

Foot of table or bed elevated 14 inches (about 15°). Patient lies head down on right side and rotates ¼ turn backward. Pillow may be placed behind from shoulder to hip. Knees should be flexed. Therapist claps with moderately cupped hand over left nipple area. In females with breast developed or tenderness, use cupped hand with heel of hand under armpit and fingers extending forward beneath the breast.

(d)

Foot of table or bed elevated 14 inches (about 15°). Patient lies head down on left side and rotates ¼ turn backward. Pillow may be placed behind from shoulder to hip. Knees should be flexed. Therapist claps over right nipple area. In females with breast development or tenderness, use cupped hand with heel of hand under armpit and fingers extending forward beneath the breast.

(e)

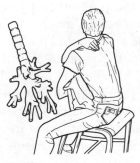

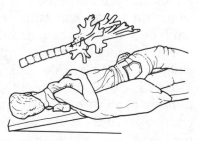

(i) Lean forward over back of chair on folded pillow at about 30° angle. Clap with cupped hand and vibrate over upper back extending fingers forward and upward.

(f)

(ii) Foot of bed elevated 10–14 inches about 15° angle. Lie on left side ¼ turn, head down (pillow behind from shoulder to hip), knees flexed. Clap and vibrate over right nipple.

allowing maximal ventilation of the lungs. Young children swallow their sputum, so the fact that none is being coughed out does not mean that no sputum is being produced.

In CF the upper lobes of the lungs are particularly prone to attack, although the reasons for this are unknown. The techniques employed in improving the strength and efficiency of the muscles of respiration and the clearing of sputum include breathing exercises (see Box 1) chest clapping with cupped hands, and sitting or lying in various positions to help mucus drainage (see Fig. 11). The paediatrician may direct the attention of the physiotherapist and the parents to an area that requires special attention, because of physical signs found on examining the chest, or on an X-ray or scan. All CF patients are taught the forced expiration technique (FET), whereby the person breathes out in short, powerful huffs. The method has been shown to result in improved lung functions, and has the great advantage of allowing older people a greater degree of freedom, since it reduces with the need for another person to help with the physiotherapy.

Inhalation of bronchodilators may be prescribed for use at or near the beginning of a physiotherapy session. Inhaled antibiotics are also taken as part of the physiotherapy session, but *at the end* (otherwise, of course, much of the antibiotic would be coughed up in the sputum and lost).

The hospital-based physiotherapist, the parents, and the child are the team that look after physiotherapy needs. In some CF clinics the physiotherapist forms the closest relationship of all with the parents. What does require discipline on the part of all, is to realize the often progressive nature of the condition, which may deteriorate despite meticulous attention to all aspects of treatment.

NUTRITIONAL AND DIETARY ASPECTS

Control of chest infections is most important in maintaining good nutrition in CF. An increase in stool frequency or steatorrhoea may herald a new chest infection rather than indicating dietary indiscretion. On the one hand, optimal nutritional care in CF may lead to a reduction in chest infections. In the face of more advanced disease, particularly

Breathing exercises

If the upper and lower airways become blocked, faulty breathing habits may develop, with poor movement of the lower chest. The over-expanded lungs may reduce the mobility of the chest wall and diaphragm. The increased effort may result in poor posture, with round shoulders and a forward position of the head. Breathing exercises improve ventilation and posture by allowing more efficient use of the diaphragm and muscles of the abdomen in breathing. Improved breathing and relaxation of the muscles of the upper chest, neck, and shoulders allow better lung function and posture.

A summary of a good breathing exercise follows.

Place one hand on the upper chest and one on the abdomen. Breathe in deeply through the nose — the abdomen should rise but the upper chest should remain still. Breathe out slowly with the lips pursed, making the sound 'pff' — this increases the pressure inside the airways and prevents them from collapsing too soon in expiration. Note that the abdomen has become flat. The out breath should take three times as long as the in breath.

The exercise described above can be done lying flat or sitting in a chair with the back well supported. If done sitting, one bends over during expiration. In the lying position, placing of a book or graded weights (anything from 1 lb to 10 lb) on the abdomen provides an extra load for the diaphragm and abdominal muscles to move and increases their strength and bulk, much as the biceps are developed using a barbell.

Other exercises include blowing bubbles, balloons, candle flames, and counting games on a single breath. Sit-ups are excellent for strengthening abdominal muscles. Lie on your back on the floor; with the arms folded across the chest, come slowly to a sitting position. Try to daily increase the number of sit-ups you are able to do before tiring.

Leg raising, push-ups, forward bends, and weight-lifting strengthen the shoulder and abdominal muscles.

The stronger all these muscles are, the easier coughing becomes. Abdominal pain from frequent or deep coughing is thus lessened. Breathing exercises are especially important in girls, who tend to have less well developed musculature.

in adolescence, anorexia may contribute to poor nutrition.

Recent improvements in the quality and type of pancreatic enzyme supplements available have resulted in a great reduction in one of the most unpleasant side-effects of CF, namely steatorrhoea. Nevertheless, dietary indiscretion may still lead to a return of frequent bulky, strong-smelling stools.

In CF, poor food absorption means that much food value is lost in the faeces. Also, tissue damage caused by the disease increases the amount of protein and energy that the body requires. Thus people with CF must have a diet that is high in protein and calories but low in fat. A number of studies have shown that most CF patients actually eat less than the recommended amounts.

The exact types of fats that we eat have been attracting attention in recent years. An analysis in London showed that most children with CF received diets with too little of the polyunsaturated, essential fatty acids (those fatty acids that the body needs but cannot manufacture for itself), which need to be taken in the diet. These fats play a role in maintaining the health of the body membranes, e.g. in the lung, and are more easily digested than most fats. Rules which seem reasonable to follow are:

(a) as a cooking oil use a pure oil produced from seeds, either soya, sunflower, or corn-oil;

(b) choose a margarine labelled 'high in polyunsaturates', e.g. one made from sunflower or soya oil;

(c) avoid hidden fats such as those in pastries, pies, burgers, milk chocolate, and crisps.

It is possible to increase the nutritional value of ingested fat in this way. Nutritionists believe that about 3 per cent of the energy requirements in CF should be taken as essential fatty acids.

Over the years there have been attempts to provide 'elemental' diets, consisting of predigested mixtures of amino-acids, thus avoiding the need for pancreatic supplements. One example that still has a few very faithful adherents is the Allan diet, consisting of a pre-digested beef serum, a glucose polymer, and medium chain triglycerides. This diet is taken either as the sole means of nutritional support or as an additive. It is expensive, and has a rather unpleasant taste. Certain patients gain weight on the diet, but none of the other benefits originally claimed for it (improved lung function or X-ray appearance) have been proved in a carefully performed study. The diet may have a role in underweight adolescents who are very conscious of their body image.

Pancreatic enzymes

Preparations of pancreatic enzymes from pigs have been used for many years to supplement the digestive enzymes of CF patients. A recent improvement in these enzyme supplements has been the introduction of enteric-coated microspheres (e.g. Pancrease®, Creon®). These microspheres resist the attack of acid in the stomach, thus allowing a much greater proportion of the supplement taken to reach the duodenum where it is needed. This means that CF patients need far smaller amounts of enzyme supplement in their diet.

One preparation now in use has an even greater effectiveness, because it is not heat-sterilized during manufacture. In theory the older, sterilized preparations are safer, but in practice, no bowel infections have been found in patients on the unsterilized supplements. On the contrary, these people have shown improved weight gain, an improvement in stool quality and a great increase in patient convenience with almost no side-effects. There are some people who are very well controlled on other pancreatic preparations, e.g. Cotazyme®; Pancrex V®; Nutrizyme®, and there is no reason for such people to change the preparations used. One formulation which should be avoided, however, is Cotazyme B®. This only contains lipase and little or no trypsin.

It has been suggested that an elegant new group of drugs, which reduce the amount of acid produced by the stomach and aid its emptying may be of use in treating CF. (Examples of these drugs are cimetidine and ranitidine.) Although such drugs are effective in treating people with peptic ulcers, it does not seem desirable to interfere with the normal working of the stomach over a very long period of time.

Recently, with more effective pancreatic supplements available, some clinics have been experimenting in allowing a far more liberal diet, balancing the number of enzyme capsules taken against the number and quality of stools and ensuring that weight gain continues to be adequate. For most people, however, some reduction in the amount of fat in the diet will probably remain necessary.

In a recent experimental trial, 12 volunteers were given a diet consisting of soya oil, amino acids, and glucose at 130 per cent of the recommended daily intake levels. The diet was given entirely by injection into a vein. Those given the treatment showed a weight gain that was still retained six months later, and had significantly fewer chest infections and improved lung function. By its nature, this study could not be performed in a controlled fashion, i.e. it was impossible to give another group other substances intravenously, for comparison. However, this emphasizes the fact that most people with CF do not get enough nutrients from their diet. There is a role for this type of treatment in people who remain persistently underweight.

Salt

There are increased salt needs in CF, particularly in hot weather. Certain children seem particularly prone to acute salt depletion and the need for extra salt should be considered in any child with CF who shows signs of lethargy. Occasionally, during a heatwave, a child may become weak or dehydrated and may need saline solution to be given intravenously. Dietary salt is often cited as a cause of high blood pressure, but in CF this is not the case, because increased salt in the sweat provides a safety mechanism.

Vitamins

Because of the malabsorption of fat in CF, the fat-soluble vitamins A, D, E, and K are taken by most people with the disease. There does not seem a good reason to challenge this practice, although the necessity of yet more tablets is inconvenient. There is evidence from blood tests that people with CF suffer from vitamin D deficiency, but the disease that results when there is such a deficiency, rickets, has never been described in CF. A group of CF adults in Birmingham who also suffered from ataxia (a disorder of balance) were shown to be vitamin E deficient, and the ataxia symptoms disappeared when vitamin E was administered.

Trace elements

Some elements, such as iron, selenium, and zinc are found in very small amounts in the body. They are necessary for certain body functions (for example iron is an integral part of haemoglobin, the molecule that transports oxygen around the blood), and must therefore be taken in the diet. No deficiencies of zinc, selenium, or iron have been found in people with CF, but work on other trace elements continues.

TREATMENT OF OTHER SYMPTOMS OF CF

Meconium ileus equivalent

Surgical treatment of meconium ileus equivalent may occasionally be necessary, but most attacks can be managed by increasing liquid intake and by administering water-attracting enemas (e.g. Gastrographin®) or drugs like acetyl cysteine (which thins the intestinal mucus). (Attempts to use the mucus-thinning properties of acetyl cysteine to treat lung complications in CF have proved fruitless, as the action of the drug was found to be too vigorous).

Rectal prolapse in infancy comes under control once the steatorrhoea is treated.

Diabetes

As mentioned earlier, the diabetes in CF is generally mild and small doses of insulin suffice to control it. There are generally some modifications needed in the diet, and a diabetic with CF would need to ensure that salt intake was adequate. We at RMCH generally share the care of diabetic CF patients with a diabetes specialist.

Varices

It was explained in Chapter 2 (p. 30) how varices or dilated veins occur at the lower end of the gullet in people with cirrhosis of the liver. People with varices must avoid taking aspirin or similar substances, as these drugs may cause bleeding. Individuals with varices may need to take vitamin K and drugs of the cimetidine group to reduce stomach acid. Occasionally, sclerosing agents may be needed. These drugs strengthen the walls of the blood vessels, thus making bleeding less likely. These are injected directly into the varices, under anaesthetic.

FERTILITY AND CF

Adults with CF often ask for counselling about fertility. Nearly all men with CF are sterile and their ejaculate contains no sperm. Nevertheless, in a small percentage of cases this is not so, and men with CF have been known to father children. Women with CF are fertile, though they may have abnormal cervical mucus and may sometimes come to infertility clinics. Some women are not well enough to be able to undertake pregnancies, but there are more than 100 instances on record of women with CF having had children. In two recorded instances the child was found to have CF too.

Pregnancy

Sadly, the cost of pregnancy is great for women with CF. Heart failure may occur, and lung function often deteriorates. In the only good study of its kind, 18 of 100 women who undertook pregnancies were dead within two years of giving birth, with 12 of them dying within six months. The chances of the baby dying within a few days of birth and of being premature were also increased in this group. Other factors that deserve consideration are the impact of the mother's shorter lifespan on the offspring and the possible inability of the mother to see to the child's daily needs. It is generally agreed that unless the disease is very mild, women with CF are best advised to avoid pregnancy.

Contraception

Oral contraceptives should be used with great care by women with CF, as they can cause blood clots in the veins. Oral contraceptives should be particularly avoided when there is liver damage (as in cirrhosis). For many women with CF, spermidical jelly in conjunction with condoms is the method of choice.

The foregoing are many of the general aspects that might be dealt with when genetic counselling in CF is given. Specific details of tests of pre-natal diagnosis are discussed in the next chapter.

4

Genetics of cystic fibrosis

The human body is made up of a huge number of individual functional units called cells. These cells are too small to be seen by the naked eye, but they can be looked at through a microscope in which they are magnified maybe fifty to one hundred times. Each cell is surrounded by an outer membrane, within which are a number of structures essential to the working of the cell. The nucleus is one of these. It is surrounded by another membrane, and contains among other things the genetic information of the cell. All the cells of an individual have the same genetic information. It is this information that is responsible for the inherited characteristics of an individual.

Body cells are continually dividing during life; in this way the body can grow and repair itself. When a cell divides, it produces two daughter cells, each of which contains the same genetic information as the parent cell. To achieve this, the parental cell genetic information is duplicated before cell division so that there are two sets of this information, one for each daughter cell. This type of cell division is known as *mitosis*.

When the cell is not dividing, the genetic material is spread throughout the nucleus. However, when the cell is about to divide, the genetic material contracts and coils up. As a result of these changes, the structures in each cell that contain the genetic material (known as *chromosomes*) can be seen much more clearly as specific structural bodies (see Fig. 12). Chromosomes are asymmetrical structures consist-

64

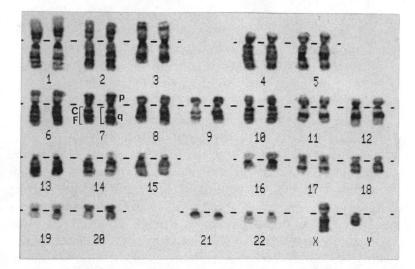

Fig. 12. The chromosomes of a normal human male individual. The banding pattern, produced with a specific stain, is characteristic of each pair of chromosomes. The CF gene is located on the long (q) arm of chromosome 7.

ing of a short (p) arm and a long (q) arm separated by a central constriction, the centromere.

Different species have different numbers of chromosomes. Humans normally have forty-six chromosomes in all the cells of their body apart from the sex cells (the eggs or the sperm). Each of these body cells is *diploid*, i.e. it carries two complete sets of genetic information. Thus the forty-six chromosomes consist of two sets of twenty-three. One chromosome set comes from the mother via the ovum (egg) and the other comes from the father via the particular sperm that fertilized the ovum. Both ovum and sperm are *haploid*, that is they carry only a single set of twenty-three chromosomes. When egg and sperm fuse in fertilization, the chromosome complement of the ensuing embryo is restored to forty-six (twenty-three pairs).

In twenty-two of these twenty-three pairs of chromosomes, members of the pair are the same in men and women. These pairs are known as the *autosomes*. The twenty-third pair comprises the sex chromosomes, X and Y. Normal women have two X chromosomes, normal men have one X chromosome and one Y. Unlike the autosome pairs, the X and Y chromosomes are functionally dissimilar. The Y chromosome is very small in comparison with the X and apparently carries very little genetic information, apart from that required to direct male sexual development.

As has already been mentioned, the ovum and the sperm only carry a single set of chromosomes. Eggs and sperm are made by a process called *meiosis*, a normal diploid cell with forty-six chromosomes divides into haploid cells containing twenty-three chromosomes each.

If meiosis simply involved one chromosome from each pair going into each haploid cell, then the maternal and paternal chromosomes would remain unchanged from generation to generation and there would be no genetic diversity. What actually happens is that during meiosis the two sets of genetic information in the cell are shuffled like two packs of cards. This process is known as recombination.

Before the cell divides in meiosis, the chromosomes join in homologous pairs. This means that chromosome 1 inherited from the mother joins up with the corresponding paternal chromosome, and likewise chromosome 2, 3, 4 etc. pair up. Random and reciprocal exchanges of genetic material then occur within each homologous pair, involving sections of genetic material from one chromosome breaking off and replacing the equivalent section on the other chromosome (see Fig. 13).

The two main chemical components of chromosomes are deoxyribonucleic acid (DNA) and proteins. It is the DNA that in its structure contains all the information needed to construct a human being from a single fertilized egg. The building blocks of DNA are chemical units of a base (a

Genetics of cystic fibrosis

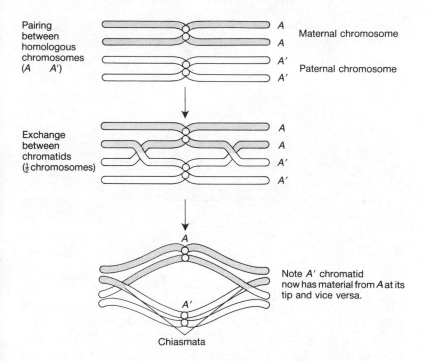

Pairing between homologous chromosomes (A   A')

A — Maternal chromosome
A
A' — Paternal chromosome
A'

Exchange between chromatids (½ chromosomes)

A
A
A'
A'

A
A'

Note A' chromatid now has material from A at its tip and vice versa.

Chiasmata

Fig. 13. Diagram to show recombination at meiosis.

nitrogen containing compound, either a purine or a pyrimidine) and a sugar molecule (deoxyribose) joined together. Many of these units are linked through phosphate molecules into a long chain (see Fig. 14(a)). The four different bases that are used in DNA are called adenine (A), guanine (G), cytosine (C), and thymine (T). These are the elements of the genetic code (the 'language' of the genetic information). The DNA in chromosomes is in the form of a double chain, the so-called 'double helix', in which the two chains are wound round each other and joined to each other by their base units (see Fig. 14(b)). The structure can be likened to a spiral staircase where the two continuous sides (sugar–phosphate back bones) are joined at regular intervals by the stairs (bases: see Fig. 14(c)). Due to differences in the sizes of the

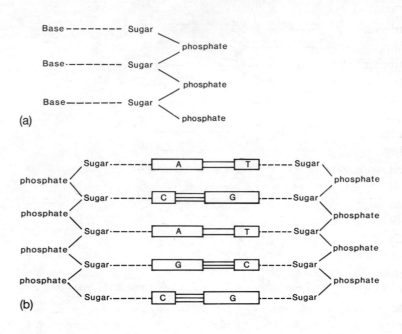

Fig. 14. The structure of DNA.
  (a) The basic DNA chain
  (b) Two DNA chains joined in a
      functional unit
  (c) The double helix in three dimensions.

individual base molecules, (adenine and guanine are bigger than cytosine and thymine), adenine can only join to thymine and guanine can only join to cytosine if the two sides of the staircase are to remain a constant distance apart.

Each DNA molecule can replicate itself, making an identical copy of its genetic information. This is what happens before mitosis, the cell division process described earlier. However, for this genetic information to be useful to the cell, it must be translated into a form that can be used by the cell machinery outside the nucleus. To achieve this the DNA has to be copied, or transcribed into another molecule, ribonucleic acid (RNA), otherwise known as messenger RNA. In turn, this messenger RNA is used as a blueprint for the translation of the genetic message into biologically useful molecules, proteins. Many thousands of different proteins are made in the one cell. Proteins can really be regarded as the primary product of genetic information and all the different proteins made in an individual are responsible for his or her uniqueness. They have a wide range of functions in the body; structural proteins are major components of muscle, skin, hair and many other tissues, while enzymes are essential parts of the body's metabolic machinery.

Since all the cells in the body arise from mitotic division of the fertilized egg, each cell carries a full complement of genetic information, i.e. 46 chromosomes. However, only a very small part of this information is being used in any one cell at any one time. In fact, much of the DNA in the chromosomes never seems to be used at all in coding for proteins. The important coding regions of the DNA are called *genes*. It is these genes that are transcribed into messenger RNA which then goes on to be the blueprint for protein manufacture, as we described above. Between genes or groups of genes are large non-coding regions of DNA. Some of these non-coding regions may have some role in controlling the activities of the genes, but the vast majority seem to have no function at all.

Cystic Fibrosis: the facts

The cells of a particular tissue or organ will have a specific set of genes in action. Hence, though the enzyme-secreting cells of the pancreas and the cells lining the respiratory system will have certain active genes in common, (that is those making products that are essential for the maintenance of any living cell), other active genes will be coding for products involved in tissue-specific functions. For example, the pancreas secretory cells will have active genes producing specific digestive enzymes to break down food, while genes coding for mucus will be switched on in many of the cells lining the respiratory tract.

It should be remembered here that each cell contains a pair of each gene, one from each parent. Genes coding for the same product can vary slightly in their precise DNA sequence from one person to the next. Where an individual has inherited identical forms (alleles) of a particular gene from both parents he is said to be *homozygous* for that gene, but if he has inherited non-identical alleles for any specific gene he is defined as *heterozygous* for that gene. The words *heterozygote* and *carrier* of a particular gene are in some cases interchangeable.

Genetic diseases are caused by abnormal genes that do not fulfil their proper function. An abnormal gene can be classed as dominant or recessive. If an abnormal gene is dominant, its abnormality is manifest even if the other gene of the pair is normal. However, when an abnormal gene is recessive, the abnormality is masked if the other gene of the pair is normal. So a person who has CF or a similar recessive hereditary disease must be homozygous for the abnormal gene, i.e. they must have inherited the abnormal gene from both parents. An individual who is heterozygous (i.e. has one normal and one abnormal gene) for a recessive hereditary disease is known as a carrier of the abnormal gene. Carriers do not have the symptoms of the disease, but may pass it on to their offspring.

The combination of all the different genes that an indi-

70

Genetics of cystic fibrosis

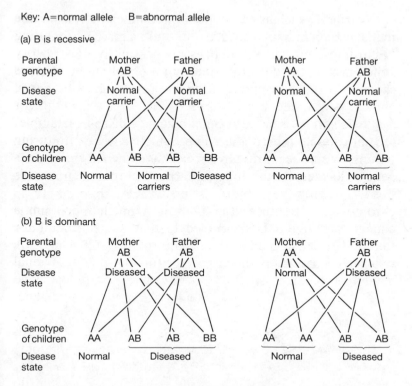

Fig. 15. Diagram to illustrate dominant and recessive inheritance.

vidual has are known as his or her genotype. Simple inheritance patterns of dominant and recessive genes are illustrated in Fig. 15.

Both dominant and recessive diseases can be subdivided into autosomal and sex-linked conditions, which are coded for by genes located on the autosomes or on the sex chromosomes, respectively. The known inheritance pattern of the CF gene, derived from the study of many affected families, shows that equal numbers of male and female CF children are born to healthy parents. From this pattern it is clear that the CF gene must be autosomal and not sex-linked. Recessive diseases coded for by a gene on the X chromosome, such as haemophilia, are much more common in males than in females. This is because a male has only one X chromosome and so there is no possibility of a normal gene masking the defective one. For a female to be affected she would have to carry the same defect on both her X chromosomes, necessarily a rare event.

Cystic fibrosis is an autosomal recessive disease, i.e. affected individuals inherit the same defective gene from both parents. Very recent research work has shown us that the CF gene is located on the long (q) arm of chromosome 7 (see Fig. 12). However, there is no visible abnormality in chromosome structure; the fault is a much more subtle change within the DNA molecule that has not yet been found. The classical inheritance pattern of the CF gene from two carrier parents is shown in Fig. 16.

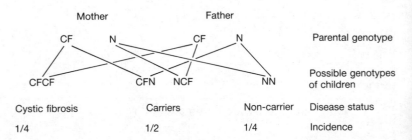

Fig. 16. Inheritance of the CF gene from two carrier parents. CF = CF gene, N = normal gene.

FREQUENCY OF CF

As has already been mentioned, CF is the most common potentially lethal autosomal recessive disease among Caucasians (white Indo-Europeans). The condition is excessively rare among Chinese races and in African Negroes. The incidence of CF among Negroes in Washington DC was found to correspond with the degree of interbreeding with whites. CF definitely occurs in natives of many Middle Eastern countries and in Pakistan. In Caucasian races, however, the CF carrier frequency is about one in 22 individuals, and one baby in around 2000 live births has the disease.

How can we explain the high frequency of CF if 98 per cent of adult males with the disorder are sterile, and until very recently females with CF were not growing up to have children?

(a) Heterozygote advantage

Most doctors and scientists believe that the high CF gene frequency is due to some heterozygote advantage. That is, carriers of the CF gene (those with one CF gene and one normal gene) have a higher reproductive input into the population than non-carriers. This could be because more CF carriers reach child-producing age, or because CF carriers have more children than non-carriers. The overall effect is that the CF gene is reintroduced into the population in each generation at a slightly higher frequency than its normal counterpart. Heterozygote advantage is still only a theory, i.e. it has not been proved. Explanations of the causes of heterozygote advantage are generally based on the idea of increased resistance to other potentially lethal diseases. Two such theoretical explanations are given below.

Influenza

It is possible that CF heterozygotes (carriers) are more resistant to influenza than the rest of the population. Hence, during the influenza epidemics that killed large numbers of people in the past, carriers of the CF gene were at an advantage.

Cholera

Another theory to account for CF heterozygote advantage relates to the known abnormalities in the movement of salts (particularly chloride), in and out of certain body cells and tissues in CF (see Chapter 2, p. 32, and Chapter 5, p. 97). It has been suggested that defective chloride ion transport might reduce the severity of cholera by inhibiting water loss from the intestine. Cholera is no longer an important disease in Western nations, but the CF gene frequency does not seem to be falling (although in genetic terms it may be too early for such a change to be obvious). Thus this theory, and a similar one based on resistance to tuberculosis, do not seem very attractive.

(b) New mutation

Other factors besides improved resistance to disease could be responsible for maintaining the high frequency of the CF gene in the population. To date there is no extensive experimental evidence for any of them but one possible theory is based on new mutation to the *carrier* state.

A mutation is a random alteration in the sequence of base pairs along the DNA in a gene. The alteration produces a gene that is different from either parent's gene (it may or may not be functional). A mutation may be caused by a mistake in DNA replication, or by environmental damage to the DNA that is subsequently not repaired properly. Thus it is possible that a proportion of CF genes in each generation are not inherited from a parent or parents, but are newly formed by mutation.

If the frequent occurrence of the CF gene in a population is due to new mutations, then the frequency of mutations producing the CF gene must balance the numbers of CF genes lost from the same population each generation. Since very few individuals with CF (i.e. homozygous for the CF gene) produce children, the loss of CF genes in each generation is quite large. The frequency with which mutations are known to occur in other genes is not as large as the loss of CF genes each generation, so mutation alone seems an insufficient explanation for the CF gene frequency.

(c) Reproductive compensation

One further possibility to account for maintenance of an unusually high frequency for the CF gene, before reliable diagnosis of CF was possible, was reproductive compensation. This theory suggests that families where a child has CF generally have more children, to 'compensate' for the possible death of the affected child. Two out of three of the healthy children will be carriers of the CF gene (see p. 72 of this chapter), so more CF genes are introduced into the population. In most instances where this theory has been studied in the past, the mean size of families with a CF child has been larger than that of families with no CF children. However, it is unlikely that this reproductive compensation is a major factor at the present time.

(d) Consanguinity

Consanguinity is inbreeding between genetically related members of the same family (for example brother and sister, first cousin or uncle and niece). In certain countries consanguinous marriages may play a part in increasing the incidence of what might otherwise be a rarer genetic condition (although consanguinity appears to have little effect in CF in most countries). In a few isolated communities, notably amongst Afrikaaners in Namibia, a much higher incidence of CF than expected has been found. In these instances the parents of those children affected could be traced back to common forebears, generations earlier. Some genealogies of the Afrikaaner population in Namibia, drawn up by one of the authors (M.S.) when he worked there, are shown in Fig. 17.

RISK FACTORS

What are the chances of having a child with cystic fibrosis? In the absence of a reliable method of carrier detection,

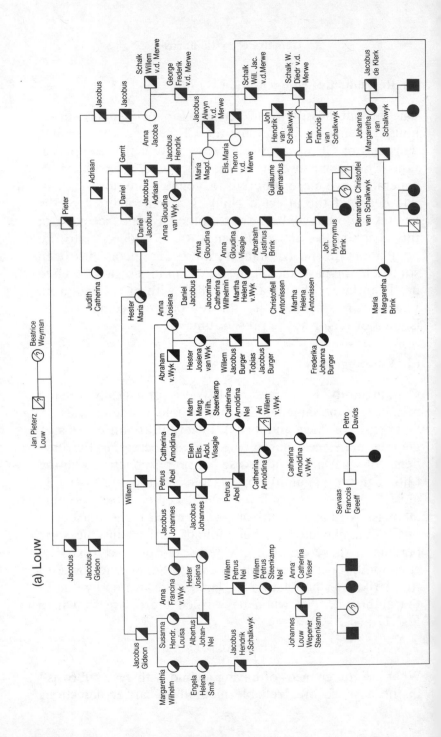

(a) Louw

(b) van der Merwe

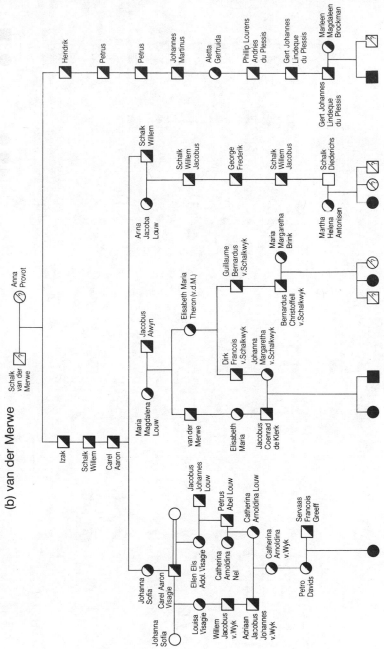

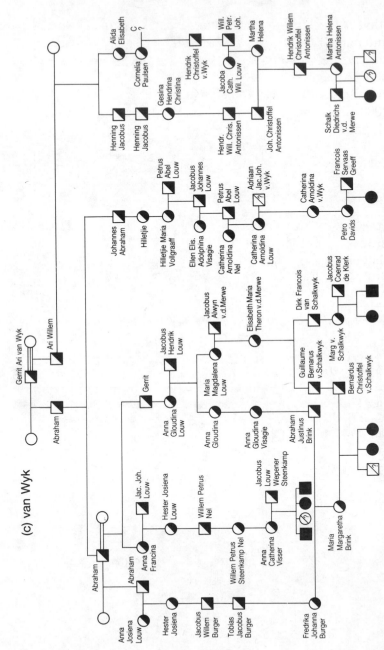

(c) van Wyk

(that is, picking up individuals who have one normal gene and one CF gene), the best one can do is to offer mathematical calculations based on the frequency of the disease and hence the estimated frequency of the carrier state. Tables 2 and 3 give information based on a disease frequency of 1 in 2000 and an estimated carrier frequency of 1 in 22 individuals in the general population.

Table 2. Chances of being a CF carrier

History	Chance
Mother has CF[a]	1/1 (i.e. definite)
Brother or sister has CF	2/3
Half-brother or sister has CF	1/2
Brother or sister has offspring with CF	1/2
No family history of CF	1/22

[a] Males with CF are generally sterile and so are not included in the table.

Fig. 17. Genealogies of some Namibian families carrying the CF gene. (a) The Louw family; (b) the van der Merwe family; (c) the van Wyk family.
Key

◯ = Female
▢ = Male
◖ = Suspected carrier female ⎫
◪ = Suspected carrier male ⎬ Assuming that the mutation giving rise to the CF gene occurred in early ancestors of the family
● = CF female
■ = CF male
⊘ = Possible carrier female
▨ = Possible carrier male
▢—◯ = Second marriage
▢═◯ = Third marriage

Table 3. Risks of having a child with CF (based on an assumption that one in twenty-two of the general population are carriers)

History	Risk
Couples with one or more CF children	1/4
Mother has CF[a]: partner has no history of CF in the family	1/44
One parent has had a child with CF: partner has no history	1/88
Brother or sister of child with CF: partner has no history	1/132
Brother or sister of parent of CF child: partner has no history	1/176
First cousins: no history of CF in the family	1/700
Unrelated couples: no history of CF in the family	1/2000

[a] Males with CF are generally sterile and so are not included in the above table.

If a couple has had a child with CF, it is clear that they must both be carriers (heterozygous). In this case, the chance that *any* of their subsequent offspring will have CF (i.e. will be homozygous for the abnormal gene) remains one in four for each pregnancy (see Fig. 16 on inheritance patterns of the CF gene). The healthy brother or sister of someone with CF has a two in three chance of being a CF carrier like his or her parents (one abnormal and one normal gene), and a one in three chance of not carrying the CF gene at all.

It should be noted here that in some genetic diseases the likelihood of carrier parents having an affected child is influenced by maternal age, birth order, or season of conception. None of these factors have any influence in CF.

Actual examples of the inheritance pattern of the CF gene are shown in the family trees of Fig. 18.

Clearly, until we have a reliable method of carrier detection, we cannot calculate more specific risk factors for any particular couple wanting advice. Chance factors are merely drawn from tables similar to those shown above. This is obviously an unsatisfactory situation. However, recent advances in CF research, using the powerful techniques of molecular biology, mean that in at least some families with CF a more scientific approach to carrier detection may be applicable. These advances will be discussed in more detail in the section on new approaches to genetic disease (Chapter 5).

HETEROZYGOTE (CARRIER) DETECTION

We saw in the previous section that at present it is difficult to make anything more than a general estimate of the chances of having a child with cystic fibrosis. A method for detecting carriers of the CF gene would allow experts to give much better advice and counselling to individuals worried about CF. If an easy and reliable test for CF carriers were available, it could be offered to any members of the public who wished to be screened. Such tests exist for other hereditary diseases (for example thalassaemia, sickle cell anaemia, and Tay–Sachs disease). Obviously the test must be voluntary, since not everyone at risk will wish to be tested.

A complex and laborious test for CF carriers would only be useful if the number of people to be screened was very small. It could be offered to people with a very high risk of being CF carriers, i.e. siblings (brothers and sisters) or to partners of people with CF, and new partners of people who have already produced children with CF.

To date a wide variety of potential CF carrier detection tests have been tried out. They include several systems in which CF heterozygotes (carriers) show values of a measured parameter intermediate between those of CF homozygotes and normal controls. These tests are considered in further detail in the basic research chapter. None of them has yet proven to be a sufficiently reliable method of heterozygote detection (but see p. 93).

Cystic Fibrosis: the facts

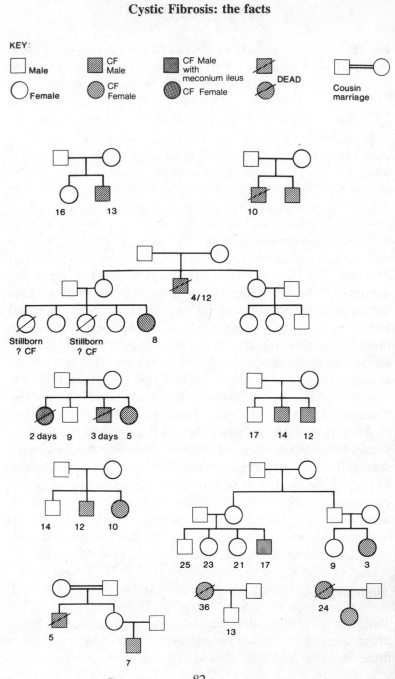

Fig. 18. Some illustrative family pedigrees. If one analysed a sufficient number of families and made allowances for those instances where both parents are carriers yet none of their children has CF, then the results would show that, where both parents are carriers, one in four of their children will be born with CF. More or less equal numbers of males and females are born with CF.

The numbers in the diagram indicate the ages of CF patients and their brothers and sisters at the time of writing, or the ages at which CF patients died (4/12 denotes four months). The chances of each non-affected brother or sister of a CF child being a CF carrier are referred to in Table 2.

METHODS OF PRE-NATAL DIAGNOSIS

The methods described below are currently used to diagnose a number of diseases before birth. Most methods of pre-natal diagnosis rely on obtaining a small sample of material from, or produced by, the unborn child (the foetus). A biochemical test or a study of the chromosomes can then be carried out on this sample. This material may be a sample of amniotic fluid (the fluid surrounding the developing embryo, which contains many cell types that have been shed by the foetus and the membranes around it), a sample of the foetal blood taken from the umbilical cord or, more recently, a small piece of the rumpled outer surface of the membranes surrounding the foetus, known as chorionic villi (see Fig. 19). The safety of this latest technique is still being evaluated. All the other procedures discussed have an acceptably low risk of interfering with the pregnancy, and have been used successfully in the pre-natal diagnosis of a variety of different genetic diseases.

Amniocentesis

This test is usually carried out 16 to 18 weeks into the pregnancy. It involves collecting a small amount of amniotic fluid from around the foetus. It was the first technique

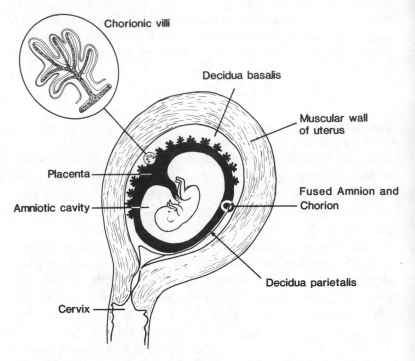

Chorionic villi

Decidua basalis

Muscular wall
of uterus

Placenta

Amniotic cavity

Fused Amnion and
Chorion

Decidua parietalis

Cervix

Fig. 19. Diagram to show the human embryo in the amniotic sac about twelve weeks into the pregnancy.

developed for pre-natal diagnosis of foetal abnormalities and is still the most frequently used. Following amniocentesis there is slightly less than one per cent increase in the chance of a miscarriage, and around a one per cent increase in the chance of a premature birth. Several tests can be carried out on this amniotic fluid. The fluid itself may have certain biochemical measurements carried out on it directly. For example, the level of a particular protein called alpha-fetoprotein that is present in amniotic fluid is characteristically found to be higher in defects of spine development such as spina bifida. There are also cells present in the amniotic fluid, and these may be grown (cultured) in the laboratory. The cultured cells can then be analysed to look for markers that are characteristic of particular diseases. One such marker is the number of chromosomes within each cell. Foetuses that have Down's syndrome (commonly known as mongolism), for example, carry three copies of chromosome 21 instead of the usual two.

Foetal blood sampling

This more recent technique involves taking a blood sample from the unborn child. The blood is most readily drawn from the vessels in the umbilical cord. The method has been used successfully in the pre-natal diagnosis of thalassaemias (defects in the structure of haemoglobin, the molecule that carries oxygen around the blood system). The test is performed after about 18 weeks of pregnancy. It carries a significant risk (perhaps ten per cent) of premature birth and a smaller risk of miscarriage (around five per cent).

Chorionic villus sampling

Amniocentesis and foetal blood sampling are only useful for diagnosis at a quite late stage of pregnancy (16 to 18 weeks). At such a late stage, termination of the pregnancy is very difficult for the mother, both physically and mentally. Chorionic villus sampling, however, can be carried out much earlier in the pregnancy (between 8 and 12 weeks after conception). The method involves the physical removal of a small piece of the rumpled outer surface (villi) of the membranes surrounding the foetus (the chorion). (Part of the chorion forms the placenta later in pregnancy: see Fig. 19.) Rapid results can be obtained with chorionic villus sampling, because tests are carried out directly on the sample itself. This is in contrast to amniocentesis, where cells from the amniotic fluid must be grown in the laboratory until enough cells have been produced for testing. Hence chorionic villus sampling provides a method of early diagnosis of hereditary disorders. The risk factors associated with this procedure are still being established but are probably nearly as low as those for amniocentesis. Allowing for the natural loss of about 4 per cent of foetuses between around 10 weeks gestation and normal term, chorionic villus sampling increases this figure to around 5–5$\frac{1}{2}$ per cent.

The basis of the procedure is to locate the position of the developing foetus and the chorionic tissue using ultrasound (see Fig. 19). Solid objects deflect very high frequency sound waves (ultrasound) passed across the abdomen and these deflections are translated into an image of the developing pregnancy on a television screen. A thin, hollow tube is then passed through the cervix (the neck of the womb) and guided to the chorion using the image on the ultrasound scan. A very small piece of chorion (about 2 mm wide) is sucked into the tube and removed for testing. The sample may also be taken through the wall of the abdomen, similar to amniocentesis. Chorion tissue is growing very rapidly at this stage in pregnancy, so the cells in the sample will be dividing rapidly. This is ideal for rapid chromosome analysis, as well as for direct investigation using the techniques of biochemistry and molecular biology.

Ultrasound

As explained in the previous section, ultrasound can be used to obtain a picture of the developing pregnancy. This image on its own can be useful in showing up certain abnormalities in the unborn child. These are generally malformations of the foetus that alter its normal appearance in an ultrasound scan, for example large-scale abnormalities of the spinal cord. Meconium ileus, the blockage of the bowel that occurs in some CF babies and was discussed in Chapter 2, may occasionally be detected by ultrasound scanning. Its role in pre-natal diagnosis is a very limited one, but it may be useful in conjunction with other tests in suggesting that a foetus may have CF. Ultrasound has the advantage of being non-invasive and so does not increase the chance of spontaneous miscarriage.

History of pre-natal diagnostic tests for CF

During the last eight years or so several proposed pre-natal diagnostic tests for CF have been publicized (some of these are discussed further in Chapter 5). However, in all cases, further clinical trials have failed to confirm the reliability of the tests.

Three proposed CF detection methods tried on amniotic fluid were:

(a) measuring the activities of some enzymes in amniotic fluid cells derived from CF foetuses after exposing these cells to certain foreign compounds;

(b) measuring the ability of CF-derived amniotic fluid cells to withstand the lethal effects of certain drugs;

(c) measuring the activities of specific enzymes made in the pancreas of the unborn child.

The current proposed pre-natal diagnostic test for CF is still under clinical trial at the time of going to press. The new test is at least based on a definite diagnostic feature of the disease. It is known that CF is associated with abnormalities in the function of the epithelial (lining) cells of exocrine glands (e.g. the pancreas, the sweat glands). Many of these cells, particularly in sweat glands, pancreas, and bronchi, have thousands of tiny folds in their surfaces, known as microvilli. Dr David Brock and his research group decided to investigate the amounts of specific enzymes, normally located in the cell membranes of these specialized microvilli, found in CF and non-CF amniotic fluids. The three enzymes being looked at are called GGTP, APM, and intestinal alkaline phosphatase. All three appear to be substantially less abundant than normal in amniotic fluids from foetuses subsequently shown to have CF.

Results of the Brock test to date seem very promising. However, while remaining optimistic, we await the outcome of further clinical trials to establish the exact reliability of the test. False positive results (i.e. results that predict CF but prove wrong) and false negative results (i.e. results that predict a normal child who proves to have CF) using this enzyme assay have recently been reported by Brock. The false positive rate was 6 per cent and the false negative rate 4.6 per cent.

Perhaps the most exciting recent development in the search for a pre-natal diagnostic test for CF has been the discovery by four separate, though communicating, research groups, of one protein and four DNA markers that are inherited with the CF gene. These markers, which are located on chromosome 7, will be discussed further in the section on new approaches to genetic disease in Chapter 5 (p. 105). Suffice it to say that though these DNA markers may not be useful individually in all cases of CF, in combination they may be of value for the pre-natal diagnosis of CF in most familes at risk. Furthermore, the markers are likely to provide handles on the CF gene itself. Once this is found pre-natal diagnosis of CF should be possible in nearly all families at risk.

GENETIC COUNSELLING IN CF

Genetic counsellors in the UK are medically qualified and may or may not specialize in genetics. The paediatrician or physician at the CF clinic may provide the counselling. When a couple or individual ask for genetic counselling there is an inference that they would wish to know the answers to certain questions. In providing these answers the counsellor will need to provide an understanding of the disorder. In the case of CF, this will include the possible ranges of severity in different affected individuals; the burden of the condition both for the affected person and the family; the types and effectiveness of the life-long treatment necessary and a word on life-expectancy.

Parents of newly diagnosed children with CF may not know all the implications of the diagnosis and will need this information to help them to exercise their options. When the illness itself has been discussed the risks of recurrence in any further children born will be mentioned and the autosomal recessive nature of CF explained.

Parents whose children are born with meconium ileus and who turn out to have CF, are in especial need of counselling. We have seen that meconium ileus in newborn children is very often associated with subsequent CF affected babies also having meconium ileus. In two cases known to the authors, children were born with meconium ileus and had to be operated on, but by the age of eight months these babies were thriving. The parents of these children found the experience of their children being born with meconium ileus extremely traumatic, and felt that CF without meconium ileus would have been preferable to meconium ileus alone. It was apparent from this reaction that the parents did not fully appreciate the long-term nature of CF, and the sacrifices and strains that it can cause. These facts were gently explained in counselling.

A risk of 1 in 4 of having another affected child, as it would be for parents of a child with CF, constitutes a high risk with the same chance of occurring as of two coins falling 'heads'. Couples who realize the magnitude of this risk may wish to discuss options open to them — until recently these included a decision to have no further children and possibly to try for adoption, occasionally a decision to take the 1 in 4 chance, and sometimes to opt for artificial insemination, using donor sperm (taking this step would reduce the chances of having an affected child from 1 in 4 to 1 in 88 if one assumes that a sperm donor with no family history of CF would have a 1 in 22 chance of being a carrier). Occasionally parents of a child with CF divorce and the genetic implications may have played a role. Their risk with new partners would again be 1 in 88 for each of them.

Although some studies have shown the parents of children with CF to be less put off having further children than parents of children with other serious hereditary diseases, the general tendency has been for the child with CF to be the last born to that couple. For several disorders (for example spina bifida or Down's syndrome) the existence of pre-natal tests for these diseases has influenced couples and encouraged them to undertake a further pregnancy in the knowledge that the presence of the disorder can be excluded or confirmed in the unborn baby. They understand that they would opt for abortion if the disorder were to be diagnosed in the foetus. Before the existence of a test for CF, in an American study, parents who had children with CF were asked what they thought about the idea of a pre-natal test to diagnose CF. The majority of parents said that they would be interested, though a number said they would not want such tests to be performed and others said they would not opt to end the pregnancy.

Of course, people differ very strongly in their views on abortion and pre-natal diagnosis in general. For couples at risk of having a child with CF, the existence of real treatment possibilities and the good chances of the child reaching adulthood in reasonable health may be strong arguments against pre-natal tests.

It is a sad fact that diagnosing CF pre-natally would not help to cure the unborn child. Pre-natal diagnosis of CF would only offer two options; abortion or birth of an affected child.

Until recently we were unable to diagnose CF prenatally so there was no option of pre-natal diagnosis with abortion of the affected foetus. Now this has changed dramatically, first with the test on amniotic fluid at 16–18 weeks described on p. 87, and still more recently tests on chorionic villus material as outlined in pp. 85–6, possible at 9 or 10 weeks. These newer tests are sufficiently accurate to be offered prospectively. The genetic counselling session has suddenly become very factual, with detailed explanation of how the testing of the DNA of the parents and affected child might prove fully, partially, or non-informative (see Fig. 20). In a fully informative situation one is able to tell which relevant part of chromosome 7 has been inherited from each parent and it would then be possible to diagnose with a high degree of accuracy whether the foetus was destined to have CF, to be a carrier, or to be free of CF genes, using tests on chorionic villus material.

In the partially informative situation one could exclude CF in DNA samples from chorionic villus material half the time. In the remaining half a 50:50 chance of CF would remain and some people would then offer Brock's test on amniotic fluid alkaline phosphatase at 17–18 weeks. This same test can be offered when tests are entirely non-informative. Brock's test sometimes gives false results in both directions; i.e. 5–10 per cent of the time when the test has predicted an affected foetus the child when born has been free of CF, and occasionally when the prediction has been of a foetus free of CF, the child has in fact been affected by the disease. As more gene probes are discovered, and eventually when the CF gene itself is found, more and more tests will prove fully informative, with full pre-natal diagnosis possible in the first three months of the pregnancy.

Present genetic counselling will discuss the need for pregnancies to be reported as soon as they are confirmed. An ultrasound scan will be arranged so that the duration of the pregnancy thus far, from the size of the early foetus, can be assessed. This allows arrangements for chorionic villus sampling at 8–10 weeks to be made.

Cystic Fibrosis: the facts

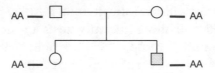

(a) Uninformative. Both parents are homozygous for band A.

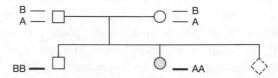

(b) Fully informative. Both parents are heterozygous for bands A and B. The CF child has inherited A bands from both parents while the non-CF child has inherited B bands from both parents. The A band is therefore linked to CF in this family. An unborn child with bands AA would have CF, with bands BB would be normal and with bands AB would be a carrier.

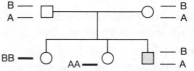

(c) Partially informative. We do not know which A and which B band in the parents is linked to the CF gene, but both sisters who are homozygous for the A or B bands, respectively, would be expected to be carriers since both the mother and the father are carrying either an A or a B band linked to the CF gene.

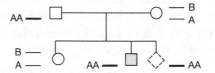

(d) Partially informative. The AB band pattern indicates a carrier while the AA band pattern has a 50 : 50 chance of indicating CF or only a carrier.

In families (c) and (d) the finding of a pattern similar to that of the boy with CF would give a 50 : 50 chance of CF in an unborn child.

Fig. 20. DNA technology applied to genetic counselling.
Key

○ = female	◉ = CF male
□ = male	◇ = unborn child
▣ = CF female	

A and B are gene probes very closely linked to the CF locus.

92

Genetics of cystic fibrosis

Couples who feel that they would wish to have pre-natal diagnosis should endeavour to have DNA from themselves and their affected child or children analysed *before* undertaking a pregnancy. This merely requires giving a small blood sample of 5–10 ml from which the DNA is extracted. If counselling occurs and tests are started with a pregnancy already under way, the laboratory may not be able to complete its work in time for the chorionic villus biopsy. It is also more difficult for the couple to think clearly about which options they would really wish to exercise. The laboratory has to drop its testing of those families without pregnancies to do the emergency work and its costs escalate.

In families where the new DNA tests prove informative it is possible to test the brothers and sisters and tell whether they are carriers. Again, in the absence of a test which could detect carriers in a spouse from the general population, some brothers and sisters would prefer not to know whether they are carriers or not. Others are very keen to be tested.

If a very recent claim is substantiated, then the gene for CF may have been located. Testing with a polymorphic probe closer to the CF locus than any tested thus far shows one band pattern almost invariably with CF-bearing chromosomes. This might enable us to offer screening for the carrier state of CF to members of the general population, especially those who marry into families with CF.

5

Research into cystic fibrosis

Perhaps this chapter would be more accurately entitled 'Basic research — which direction?' Despite nearly 40 years of research work on the changes in body chemistry (biochemistry) in cystic fibrosis, we still do not know the precise nature of the basic defect. All genetic diseases are ultimately shown up by specific biochemical changes in the body due to defective protein molecules being made (see p. 69). Further, it is not possible to logically connect together the many diverse observations on the biochemistry of CF that have been recorded over this period. Most of the biochemical changes that have been observed appear to be secondary effects of the disease. Others are seen, on further examination, to reflect normal biological variation between individuals rather than being specific to CF. In fact, the whole field of CF research is confused. It is partly because of this that progress has been disappointingly slow. It is very rare for a new observation to be made in CF research without the almost automatic subsequent appearance of several scientific papers reporting that other laboratories have been unable to reproduce the original observation. Why is this? Well, it is obviously not easy to answer such a question accurately. However, there appear to be two major contributory factors involved.

The first of these is the difficulty of doing practical research on a human disease, particularly one that affects children. Clearly the research scientists need to obtain an adequate source of human material on which to work. Their requirements must, however, be balanced against the natural unwillingness of doctors, research workers, and parents to further disturb children who are already sick, in order to obtain biological samples for purposes not directly related to treatment. As a result of this, many research projects into the biochemistry of CF have been carried out on samples from too few subjects. That is to say, the number of CF patients and normal control individuals that have been studied has been too few to rule out differences due to natural variation in the population. As a result the observations are not truly significant. When a larger population sample is examined, it is found that the factor that was proposed as being specific to people with CF also occurs in some normal individuals, and further, is not found in all CF patients.

The second difficulty relates to the pressing medical need to find the basic defect in CF, or at least to find reliable methods for detecting and treating the disease. As a result of this pressure, many methods for detecting CF that showed promise in the laboratory have been prematurely published and offered to medical practitioners. Doctors and research scientists alike have been guilty of underestimating the difficulties of transferring a test from the laboratory to hospital or clinic. An elaborate laboratory technique might well be totally impractical for routine use. In a field such as CF research, the experimental scientist must be acutely aware of these potential problems and make sure his or her data is absolutely reliable before approaching the clinical situation. As stated previously, it is essential for new tests to be applied to a large number of patients and controls in order to establish their reproducibility. But it is equally important that the techniques used in the test are clearly explained. A large amount of research time, energy, and money is wasted trying to repeat poorly described or merely unreliable tests. Obviously a test for CF that can only be carried out in one laboratory is not a useful one.

Yet another contributory reason for the slow advance of CF research science is that, unlike for many other human diseases, there are no natural animal models on which research into the disease can be carried out. Many faults in the human genetic material are also found in the genetic material of other animals, and have similar effects. Thus the diseases that these faults cause in humans can be reproduced in colonies of laboratory rats or other animals. Studies on these animals can then provide valuable information about the human disease. Unfortunately no laboratory animals have a naturally occurring disease that resembles CF.

At a fairly basic level CF research can be divided into three main areas, namely secretions, blood serum, and cells. Of course, these areas may well be overlapping in terms of biochemical causes and effects. For purposes of clarity though, they will be considered separately. In all cases the basic approach of research work has been to examine material from people with CF and to try and find factors that are common to all CF patients but are not found in healthy individuals or in other diseases. Alternatively, factors that are present in healthy individuals may be absent from CF patients.

Secretions

Three readily available secretions from CF patients have been analysed extensively, namely mucus, sweat, and saliva.

Mucus

Early clinical descriptions of CF noted that the mucus in sputum, meconium, and duodenal contents was more viscous than normal. CF mucus was said to be thicker, more sticky, and to have a greater tendency to form strands than did normal mucus. However, it seems that the abnormalities in CF mucus that were reported in early work may simply be secondary effects of contamination of the mucus by large quantities of bacteria, white blood cells, and general debris resulting from lung infection. A broad range of studies on the biochemical constituents of mucus have failed to produce consistent evidence for any abnormalities in the mucus itself.

Sweat

Sweat, as has already been discussed, provides one of the major clinical markers for CF, namely there are unusually high concentrations of simple charged molecules (ions) such as sodium (Na^+) and chloride (Cl^-) in the sweat. If a clue could be found as to the mechanism responsible for this abnormality in the sweat, it could be of crucial importance in understanding the basic defect in CF. Under normal conditions epithelial cells (cells that line the sweat ducts) reabsorb ions from the sweat passing through the ducts. When sweat is produced in the secretory part of the sweat gland, it contains the same concentration of ions as do most body fluids. Removal of ions by these specialized epithelial cells reduces the ion concentration in the sweat to much lower concentrations, and thus conserves the body's supply of ions. There has been convincing evidence recently that rates of sodium and chloride reabsorption are lower than normal in sweat glands of CF patients. The effect is most marked for chloride. It appears that in CF there is a defect in the epithelial cells of the sweat ducts and airway epithelia, which reduces the ability of these cells to transport chloride across the cell membrane. This could result in less chloride being reabsorbed from the sweat and would explain the characteristic increase in sweat salt found in CF. There have also been some suggestions, based on experimental systems, that CF sweat may contain factors inhibiting some of the normal movements of sodium ions in and out of cells. This suggestion will be discussed further in the section on tissue culture systems.

Saliva

It is questionable whether saliva from CF patients does show any abnormality associated with the disease. However, since it is a readily available material it has been the subject of several research projects. Unfortunately, none of these have yielded important information on differences in saliva bio-chemistry between CF patients and controls. One observation on CF saliva, which fits in well with the results of work on CF blood serum, is its apparent ability to interfere with the transport of sodium ions across membranes.

Blood serum

Probably the most popular human material for CF research has been blood serum (the clear fluid that can be removed after the blood has been clotted outside the body). As a result the research literature on CF serum is abundant. Several properties that have apparent genuine significance have been recorded in serum from CF patients or from carriers. These include factors specific to CF serum; factors present in normal serum that are lacking from CF serum; and normal serum constituents that are in some way abnormal in CF serum. To date, the first of these categories have provided the most interesting information on the biochemistry of CF. An important point that has often been overlooked in many of these studies is the possible effect of CF chest infections and their treatment on the biochemistry of the blood. For example, frequent courses of antibiotics and various drug therapies may have effects on the serum of CF patients. These effects may mask or alter the disease process. The disease itself may also induce secondary changes in the serum. Studies of obligate carriers (parents of CF patients) may allow observations of relevance to the basic genetic defect to be distinguished from these therapeutic or disease side effects.

Several factors have been found that are specific to serum from CF patients, and these are discussed below.

(i) Ciliary dyskinesis factor

Cilia are tiny hair-like protrusions from the epithelial cells lining the bronchial tubes (they are also found in other parts

98

of the body). These cilia have a sychronized wave motion, rather like the movements of a sea anenome's tentacles. The wave motion helps remove mucus, small particles of dirt and cell debris from the lungs by wafting them up through the trachea (windpipe) and out of the lungs.

A factor from CF serum that could disrupt this action of the cilia in rabbit tracheae was discovered in 1967. The same factor (known as ciliary dyskinesis factor) was found to be present in the serum of most parents with CF children (i.e. CF carriers). It was also found rarely among people with no history of CF, but at a frequency that could be explained by assuming that these were undiagnosed CF carriers.

Since this discovery, a wide variety of biological assay (measurement) systems have been developed to try and use this action of CF serum on cilia as a basis for a test for CF or CF carriers. In these systems various tissues that have been found to be sensitive to the ciliary dyskinesis factor have been used. Examples include the ciliated cells of hamster and guinea pig tracheae, ciliary activity in freshwater mussels and oysters, and the bacterium *Proteus vulgaris*. To date none of these systems has proved reliable. (For example, there are seasonal variations in the way that oysters and mussels react to the ciliary dyskinesis factor.)

There are two other major drawbacks to the use of ciliary dyskinesis factor as a diagnostic test for CF. One is the fact that different effects are found using the same methods in different laboratories. The other is that the factor is not specific enough: it has also been found in some patients with asthma or chronic bronchitis.

Despite numerous attempts to purify the ciliary dyskinesis factor, all efforts to date have been unsuccessful and its precise nature is not known. Possibly more than one factor is responsible for the disruptive action of CF serum on cilia — this may partly account for the difficulties in purifying it. It is also interesting to note that while the cilia of a number of species (both vertebrate and invertebrate) are affected by ciliary dyskinesis factor, the human cilia that have been studied are not. This means that the poor clearance of secretions from the lungs in CF cannot be blamed on uncoordinated ciliary beating.

(ii) 'The CF protein'

Another factor found in CF serum that has generated a large amount of experimental data and some confusion is a specific protein, called the 'CF protein' in the original reports.

The 'CF protein' was found in the vast majority of CF patients and carriers of the gene but only in very few normal controls, at a frequency which could be accounted for by undiagnosed carriers. Unfortunately the techniques available for detection of the CF protein are very demanding, and this may account for lack of success in reproducing the original observations in a number of other laboratories. The CF protein remains an elusive molecule.

Several attempts have been made to use the CF protein in the detection of CF carriers. Some of the methods involve trying to make a clinically useful antibody to the CF protein.

Antibodies are part of the body's defence system against foreign substances (antigens). They are produced by the body to specifically react with and destroy or inactivate particular antigens. The body's defence mechanism against foreign substances is called the *immune system*. It is an extremely complex system composed of many different interacting cells and molecules. The aim of the immune system is to recognize foreign substances and then trigger a reaction (the immune response) to them, leading ultimately to their inactivation.

The natural immune response of animals can be exploited to produce medically and biologically useful antibodies. The procedure involves injecting purified samples of a substance of interest (usually a protein) into a laboratory animal. The animal then produces antibodies that specifically bind to and inactivate that protein (without causing any harm to the animal itself). Thus, by injecting small amounts of purified CF protein into a laboratory animal, it should be possible to produce an antibody to it. Recently, a research group has succeeded in producing a reliable antibody specific to the CF protein. Work is continuing to establish the clinical usefulness of this antibody.

(iii) Sodium transport inhibitor

A third factor specific to CF serum that has received much attention is a sodium transport inhibitor. Clearly this fits in well with reports of a similar factor in CF saliva. The question of abnormalities in sodium transport in CF will be considered further in the section on CF cell biology (p. 102).

CF CELLS IN TISSUE CULTURE AND RELATED STUDIES

Individual cells from some human tissues can be maintained in the laboratory, alive and actively dividing, for long periods of time. The cells are kept bathed in a nutrient medium, a solution of the specific nutrients needed for those particular cells. This procedure of growing cells is known as tissue culture. Many CF researchers have worked with cultures of skin fibroblast cells or certain blood cells. (Skin is made up of a variety of cell types, of which the fibroblasts are the easiest to grow in culture.) The blood cells used in CF studies have either been erythrocytes (red blood cells) or lymphocytes (cells involved in the immune system). Neither of these cell types can be maintained in culture for long periods but lymphocytes may be turned into 'immortal' cell lines (i.e. groups of cells that will go on dividing indefinitely) by transforming them with specific viruses. It should be reiterated here that there is no evidence that either skin fibroblast cells or blood cells function abnormally in people with CF. Though, of course, all cells in the body carry the defective CF gene it may only be active in specific cell types. Considerable research efforts are currently going into attempts to culture the specific cell types which are likely to have active CF genes. However, there are two areas of CF research on other cell culture systems that deserve further description, namely ion transport studies and studies on glycoprotein synthesis and degradation.

(a) Ion transport

In order for the metabolic machinery of a cell to function efficiently, the biochemical composition of the fluid within the cells must be maintained within narrow limits. The composition of this intracellular fluid may be different from that of the fluid surrounding the cell. Since the membrane around the cell is permeable to liquids and small molecules (i.e. they can pass freely across it), there is a natural tendency for the internal environment of the cell to adjust to the composition of the body fluid surrounding it. In order to maintain the internal environment, the cell has elaborate mechanisms to pump out unwanted molecules while pumping in necessary ones. These pumps are known as the *ion transport systems* of the cell, since the majority of molecules moved are simple charged molecules (ions) such as sodium, calcium, potassium, magnesium, chloride and bicarbonate.

We have already seen that in CF the ion transport systems in the sweat gland function abnormally. It therefore seems possible that a defect in the cell's ion transport system may be the basic problem in CF. Hence, not surprisingly, the cellular ion transport systems of sodium and calcium have been the subject of numerous investigations. However, a single ion transport system cannot be investigated in isolation. Many ion movements in or out of the cell, such as those of sodium and calcium, are closely interrelated. Thus a primary defect in the transport of one ion could also affect the movement of others.

Some research work suggested that sodium ion uptake appeared to be defective in cultures of CF skin fibroblast cells. It was thought that a similar abnormality in sodium ion reabsorption by epithelial cells in the walls of the CF sweat ducts could explain the high concentrations of ions in the sweat of CF patients. More recent convincing data, already discussed in the section on CF sweat research, shows that the major defect in epithelial cells is probably one of chloride ion rather than sodium ion transport.

Other ion transport mechanisms that have been reported to be defective in CF are those involved in movements of calcium across the cell membrane. Initial reasoning for these studies on calcium ions transport was twofold. First, CF glycoprotein-rich secretions (e.g. mucus: see next section for description of glycoproteins) had been observed to contain abnormally high levels of calcium as well as sodium. Second, it was thought that high levels of calcium, which could lead to aggregation of mucous glycoproteins, might increase the viscosity of these secretions. Though again in this area of CF research early data has proven to be controversial, there is an accumulation of apparently convincing evidence that there may be an abnormality in one specific calcium ion transport system in CF. This defect has been observed in cultures of skin fibroblasts and erythrocytes. Clearly further work will have to be carried out to find out whether the defect is present in the secretory cells that seem to show a primary involvement in CF.

Research into ion transport defects using cell cultures from CF patients has produced some interesting results. But there are several major problems still to be resolved in this area of research. More work on ion transport in normal cells may resolve these questions.

(b) Glycoprotein biosynthesis and degradation

Glycoproteins are large, complex biological molecules consisting of carbohydrate units attached to a protein backbone. (Figure 21.) The precise properties of each glycoprotein are

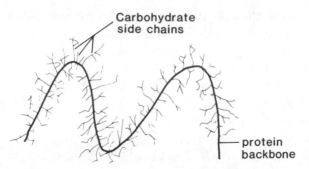

Fig. 21. Diagram of a mucous glycoprotein.

determined by the type and arrangement of the sugars in the carbohydrate portion of the molecule. The biological functions of glycoproteins are many and diverse, but historically the main glycoproteins of interest in CF have been those in mucus. This is because early research suggested that mucous glycoproteins were abnormal in CF. The enzymes involved in both building up and breaking down glycoproteins have been studied extensively in CF. Results of these studies have to date been inconsistent and contradictory, so we shall here only outline the processes involved and briefly comment on the work.

Glycoproteins are made in the cell by a group of enzymes known as glycosyl transferases. These enzymes are responsible for attaching sugar or carbohydrate groups into the protein backbone of the molecule. Different glycosyl transferases are needed to attach different sugars or groups of sugars to the protein chain. Unfortunately, these enzymes are difficult to study because they are extremely unstable. Not surprisingly therefore, the results of the different studies of glycosyl transferases in CF are totally inconsistent. It does not seem justified to explore these contradictory findings further here.

The inconsistency of research results may be due to the existence of many different types of glycosyl transferase, each with its own unique properties. Useful information relating to these enzymes in CF may have to await further developments in our understanding of the normal functioning of glycosyl transferases.

Breakdown of glycoproteins is carried out mainly by enzymes called lysosomal hydrolases. These enzymes break the biochemical linkages between carbohydrates or sugars and the protein backbones of the glycoproteins. Lysosomal hydrolases are stored, when not being used, in small capsules in the cell known as lysosomes — hence the general name of the enzymes. As with the glycosyl transferases there are a variety of different lysosomal hydrolases, each one able to break the linkage between one sugar unit and a protein, or a link between two sugars.

Many of these enzymes have been studied intensively in CF cells or body fluids. Considerable publicity has been given to research work suggesting that in cultures of CF skin fibroblasts, lysosomal hydrolases leak out of the cells and are easily inactivated by heat. However, no consistent findings have been established, and studies in CF lysosomal hydrolases will not be considered further here. It is, however, worth mentioning that some of the inconsistency in results in this area of research may be due to natural variation in the activity of these enzymes, both between different individuals, in the same individual at different times, and as a result of tissue culture conditions. Some of these factors may not have been taken fully into account in CF studies to date.

NEW APPROACHES TO GENETIC DISEASE[a]

Advances in the field of molecular biology (the explanation of biological processes in terms of molecules) over the last 10 years have opened up a whole new research area into human genetic diseases. Recombinant DNA technology, or 'The

[a] The research work discussed in this section involves many complex concepts and is difficult to explain in simple terms. The passages in this section that are in normal-sized type give a basic outline of this work. The sections in smaller type give more details for those who wish to know more about the subject.

New Genetics' as it is sometimes called, involves trying to detect the basic defects that cause hereditary diseases. The sites of these defects are within the genetic material itself, in the structure of the DNA that makes up the chromosomes. The research techniques involved are extremely effective and will, in due course, undoubtedly play a major role in our understanding of the whole of human genetics. Already significant advances have been made in this area of research.

We saw in Chapter 4 that each chromosome contains a large number of genes, sections of the DNA that carry the information for making a particular protein or protein subunit. We also learnt that a hereditary disease like CF is caused by a defect in one of these genes.

The unique character of each gene is given by the sequence of nucleotide bases along the section of DNA that makes up the gene (see Fig. 14 for DNA structure). If this sequence of bases is changed in some way, then the gene may function abnormally or cease to function altogether. The aim of recombinant DNA technology is to detect these changes of base sequence within a gene. Some of the techniques used to do this are outlined below.

To date two main methods of recombinant DNA technology have been used with greatest success in the study of human genetic diseases. One involves direct analysis of the gene concerned. The other method involves indirect association of the gene coding for a particular disease with another known piece of DNA physically and genetically linked to it (i.e. if two genes are located on the same stretch of DNA sufficiently close to each other, then the study of the behaviour of one gene at cell division may provide information on the likely behaviour of the other). These two approaches are considered below.

Direct analysis of a gene

In order to study a gene or group of genes (gene family) in detail, the gene of interest has to be isolated from the total

genetic material. This is feasible if we can identify the protein that is coded for by that gene or gene family. (An
example of a genetic disease where the gene product has
been identified is thalassaemia, a hereditary blood disease.
Thalassaemia is caused by abnormalities in haemoglobin,
the protein that carries oxygen around the blood system.)
Once the protein produced by the gene has been isolated,
researchers can use it to isolate the original gene from the
total genetic material.

One of the most successful applications of direct gene analysis
relates to thalassaemia, the hereditary blood disease mentioned
above. Haemoglobin, the molecule affected in thalassaemia, is a
large and complex protein made up of several subunits. Different
genes code for different subunits. This is reflected in the fact that
there are several distinct forms of thalassaemia, caused by defects
in each of the genes. The group of genes that code for haemoglobin is collectively known as the haemoglobin gene family.

Haemoglobin protein occurs in large quantities in red blood
cells, so for thalassaemia it was relatively easy to isolate the gene
product. The haemoglobin was used to isolate the messenger RNA
(mRNA) molecules coding for it (for an explanation of mRNA see
Chapter 4, p. 69). From the mRNA, researchers were able to use
purified enzymes to make the DNA sequence corresponding to the
messenger RNA. The artificially constructed DNA could then be
used to 'fish out' the matching DNA sequence of the natural gene
from the total DNA.

Unfortunately this direct approach to gene analysis cannot
yet be applied to the study of cystic fibrosis. We do not know
the primary gene defect and so have no gene product as a
starting point for the study.

Indirect analysis of a gene

At various locations throughout the human genetic material
(the genome) there exist what are known as polymorphic
sites. The sequence of bases on the DNA at these sites varies
from individual to individual. These polymorphisms can be

detected within the total cellular DNA by the use of DNA 'probe' molecules specific for each polymorphism. Polymorphic sites thus make good 'markers' within the genetic material. They occur sufficiently frequently for there to exist several by chance within close proximity to any gene coding for a hereditary disease. These genetic markers can be used to indirectly study and locate genes that code for hereditary diseases.

The polymorphic sites can be detected by a class of enzymes called restriction endonucleases. These enzymes recognize particular combinations of nucleotide sequence within the DNA and cleave the DNA at their 'recognition sites'. If the nucleotide sequence at one of these 'recognition sites' is altered the enzyme will no longer recognize it and so the DNA will not be cut. This natural variation in nucleotide sequence has thus caused a 'restriction fragment length polymorphism' (RFLP) since it has caused one restriction endonuclease to produce different length DNA fragments in different people. The DNA probes that are used to identify RFLPs in the living cell are segments of DNA that are complementary (i.e. will combine with) all or part of the DNA sequence of interest.

It is likely that any human gene will have, somewhere in the neighbouring DNA, one or more of these polymorphic markers. If a marker is closely linked to a particular gene in physical terms (that is, in terms of linear distance along the DNA molecule) then it is probable that at each generation the gene concerned and the marker will be inherited together. If a marker is not close to the particular gene on the chromosome, then when gametes (eggs or sperm) are formed by meiosis, the marker and the gene may become separated during recombination. (See Chapter 4, p. 66, for description of recombination.) The closer a marker is to the gene of interest, the more likely it is that gene and marker will remain linked over several generations.

Using the probes (mentioned above) for polymorphic markers, it is possible to look for linkage between a marker and the gene for a particular disease, even when the precise location of the gene is not known. Researchers will try probes for many markers, and look for their recurrence over several generations in a family that is known to carry the gene for the disease of interest. By chance a linkage may be found between the abnormal gene and one or more poly-morphic markers. That is, within any one family all indi-viduals who have the disease will have one form of the polymorphism while all those who are unaffected will have the other form. In the case of a recessive disease carriers will have both forms of the polymorphism.

Once a link between the affected gene and a marker has been found, then by a slow and laborious process regions of DNA neighbouring the marker can be analysed in an attempt to find the gene itself. However, a reliable polymor-phic marker probe closely linked to a genetic disease can in itself be valuable for genetic counselling, even if the gene itself has not been identified. If a family has a known poly-morphic marker associated with the abnormal gene, then the marker can be used for pre-natal diagnosis in that family. It can also sometimes be used to find out which individuals in the family are carriers of the gene (see Fig. 20).

An example of a clinical situation where the RFLP approach has already proved useful is in Duchenne muscular dystrophy (DMD). Since the disease is known from its inheritance pattern to be coded for by a gene located on the X-chromosome (X-linked) studies only had to include markers known to be localized on the X-chromosome. There are now about half a dozen probes linked to DMD that are in routine clinical use.

In the case of autosomal genetic diseases (i.e. non sex-linked ones) finding a linkage between a marker and the disease is usually a total shot in the dark, particularly where there is no information on the chromosomal location of the disease. It should be added that to have any reasonable likelihood of success in such a blind study, a huge number of hours of research must be expended, since the outcome of the project is based on chance alone.

Exclusion mapping and the discovery of CF markers

For the past few years, the indirect approach described above has been applied to try and establish a close linkage between the CF gene and a polymorphic marker or another known gene. Several research groups in England, Canada, and North America, who have established large DNA banks from three generations of CF families, have collaborated to test out any new marker probe or probe for a structural gene. For a long time this research failed to find a link between any probe tested and the CF gene. The research was not wasted, however, because the evidence that certain markers were definitely *not* linked to the CF gene meant that there were fewer areas where the gene *could* be located. (This process of elimination is called exclusion mapping.)

Finally in the summer of 1985, a research group hinted that they had found a marker linked to CF. By the end of November 1985 several research groups had published data on five probes apparently linked to the CF gene. These probes have finally provided us with a handle on the CF gene, though it may still take a great deal of research time and effort for molecular biologists to actually isolate the gene itself.

Two of the probes that have been found are for known genes, with functions apparently unrelated to CF. The other three probes are for polymorphic markers (RFLPs). All the markers found are on the long (q) arm of chromosome 7. Some of them will prove useful in the genetic counselling of certain families carrying the CF gene.

It is not yet known how close the polymorphic markers are to the CF gene itself though evidence is that they are very close. As we have already seen, the closer a marker is to the gene of interest, the more likely it is that gene and marker will remain linked over several generations. Thus a marker that is very close to the CF gene is more useful than one that is further away, since there is less chance of the marker and the CF gene becoming separated, so causing errors in diagnosis. Further research is already producing more CF gene markers, some of them are likely to be closer to the CF gene than any found so far.

At the start of this section it was stated that the sequence of nucleotide bases at a polymorphic site varied from individual to individual. For a particular polymorphic site to be useful in genetic counselling, the particular variant that is being used as a marker must be one that occurs in a reasonable percentage of the population. For example, a marker probe for a variation that is found in only 5 per cent of the population will be much less useful than a probe for a marker found in 40 per cent of the population.

Use of the marker probes linked to the CF gene

Each polymorphic marker probe linked to the CF gene may be used in tests that can be carried out on DNA derived from any tissue as well as from blood cells. For example, in a pre-natal test, cells from the chorionic villi or from amniotic fluid may be used (see Chapter 4). The total DNA in these cells, including that from chromosome 7 (which carries the CF gene) is digested into small pieces using certain specific enzymes and tested with the probes.

The chemical reactions that occur give rise to specific patterns of bands corresponding to pieces of DNA of different sizes. These band patterns can then be compared in the person with CF, his or her parents, brothers and sisters, or with the patterns of an unborn child in the same family. If any one marker probe produces only a single band in an individual, it means that the DNA on both his or her chromosome 7, contains the same form of that particular marker (the person is homozygous for that marker). When two or more bands are seen, the two chromosome 7 contain different forms of the marker and the person is heterozygous for that marker. (These band patterns do not directly relate to whether the person has zero, one (carrier) or two (affected) CF genes.)

111

The examples illustrated in Fig. 20 (p. 92) show some sample test results.

As has already been mentioned, because one is not dealing with the CF gene itself but with linked DNA marker probes, there is a built-in error rate, which depends on the frequency with which the linked probe is separated from the CF gene during egg or sperm formation (see Chapter 4). For the closest of the linked probes, information at the time of writing suggests that such separation may occur fairly rarely, probably in about one to two per cent of cases.

Couples wishing to make use of such tests, when they become readily available, should seek careful preliminary counselling. A full discussion is needed of the dangers of the techniques used in obtaining chorionic villus material. If the possibility exists of only partially informative results being obtained, then this must be made clear. The DNA from relevant family members should be tested before a pregnancy is under way, and the couple need to have their own preferred course of action very clear in their minds before undertaking such a test during pregnancy. Also, since no pre-natal treatment is available for CF, there would be no point in undergoing a test if the couple did not intend to end the pregnancy, should the test diagnose CF in the unborn child. These points have already been elaborated in the section on genetic counselling but bear repeating.

GENE THERAPY

There has been much talk recently about the chances of correcting genetic diseases by replacing the defective gene in the cells of a sick patient with a normal gene that functions correctly. In principle this could be achieved by inserting a functional gene into a specific tissue in an affected individual. If the genetic disease is caused by the lack of a particular protein, then insertion of a functional gene should theoretically correct the disease. This procedure is by no means as simple as it sounds — there are a range of major technical problems to overcome. However, there has been some recent success in correcting basic genetic defects in experimental animal models. It remains to be seen whether similar success will be achieved in human gene therapy.

Gene therapy could also perhaps be achieved by inserting the new gene into the embryo at a very early stage of development. At present, we do not have the technical capabilities to successfully perform such an operation, nor do we understand many of the critical factors for success.

In conclusion then, gene therapy is unlikely to be relevant in CF in the near future. In fact, until we can identify the CF gene, such therapy cannot even be envisaged.

6

Organizations concerned with cystic fibrosis

(A) THE CYSTIC FIBROSIS RESEARCH TRUST

The Cystic Fibrosis (CF) Research Trust was founded in 1964 by the late John Panchaud, an international business-man whose daughter had CF. Together with Dr Archie Norman (Consultant Physician to John Panchaud's daughter) and Consultant Paediatrician Dr David Lawson, John Panchaud set up the CF Trust in part of his own offices in the City of London.

The objectives of the trust today are the same as they were when it was founded:

1. To finance research in order to find a complete cure for cystic fibrosis, and in the meantime, to improve current methods of treatment.

2. To form regions, branches, and groups throughout the United Kingdom, for the purpose of helping and advising parents about the everyday problems of caring for CF children.

3. To educate the public about the disease and, through wider knowledge, to help promote earlier diagnosis.

The Trust raises funds continuously for CF research, through a few national events such as the annual 'CF week' and by the local activities of its regional groups and branches. In fact, since its foundation, the Trust has pro-vided over three and a half million pounds towards its objectives. A research and medical advisory committee,

114

consisting of members of the medical and scientific community, advise on how the Trust can best spend its resources.

The CF Trust's association with local groups is strong. They depend on regional branches and groups for the majority of their income; on the other hand they act as an information source for branches. The Trust produces a valuable regional and branch group manual. This booklet covers topics as wide-ranging as how to form and run the branch or group; the officers needed and how meetings should be organized; efficiency in fund-raising activities; publicity for the Trust through local newspapers, radio, and television; and government grants available to CF patients and their families.

(B) ASSOCIATION OF CYSTIC FIBROSIS ADULTS (UNITED KINGDOM)

The aims and objectives of this association are:

1. To help the CF adult to lead as full and independent a life as possible.
2. To promote the exchange of information.
3. To act as a forum for improving the management of problems encountered by CF adults, both medical and otherwise.
4. To provide encouragement for all those with CF and CF families.
5. To assist wherever possible the efforts of the CF Trust.

(C) THE INTERNATIONAL CYSTIC FIBROSIS (MUCOVISCIDOSIS) ASSOCIATION

The International Cystic Fibrosis (Muscoviscidosis) Association (ICF(M)A) was also founded in 1964, on the initiative of the American and Canadian CF Foundations. This organization is an international body, with one national association representing each country. In countries where there is not yet a national CF association, individuals are elected as associate members of the ICF(M)A to represent their countries until a national association has been formed and recognized by the ICF(M)A.

A scientific and medical advisory council, composed of one member from each national association, meets once every four years. This meeting coincides with the major international CF conferences held under the auspices of the ICF(M)A, which bring together the majority of CF research scientists and a large number of CF allied professionals and lay people. In the intervals between CF congresses, a twelve-member executive carries out the functions of the ICF(M)A. This executive meets annually in parallel with the European Working Group for Cystic Fibrosis, which provides continuity in Europe between international meetings. In America the annual meetings of the CF Club of North America perform a similar function.

Together the ICF(M)A meetings have provided an international forum for the discussion of the personal, organizational, social, and technical problems of CF. Through this organization, the well-established associations have been able to provide help and guidance to new national associations in the process of setting up. This advice has always tried to take into account the different cultural environments operative in different countries. Key factors here are, for example, the level of involvement of the State in medical and social services and research facilities; variations in national wealth and economic priorities in health care; and attitudes to charities, their organizations, and fund-raising activities both within government and in the community at large.

Within these constraints the purposes of the ICF(M)A, in common with those of its affiliated national associations are as follows:

1. The furtherance of the interests of children and adults who have cystic fibrosis. The improvement of medical care

available to these people and of the psychological and social care available to them and their families.

2. The stimulation, support, and advancement of research into the nature, cause, prevention, treatment, alleviation, and cure of cystic fibrosis.

3. The coordination of information services and the interchange of information on all phases of cystic fibrosis.

4. To assist in the formation of national associations devoted to cystic fibrosis, where they are required but do not yet exist.

5. The holding of meetings of representatives of government agencies, organizations, and individuals interested in the prevention, treatment, and cure of cystic fibrosis.

There are now some thirty countries whose national CF organizations are members of ICF(M)A and about half a dozen others with associate membership. The full addresses of all these associations (correct as of April 1987) are given in Appendix 1.

APPENDIX 1

Officers of the International Cystic Fibrosis (Mucoviscidosis) Association

President: Mrs Inge Saxon-Mills, Samil, Via Gerano 5, 00156 Rome, Italy.

Immediate Past President: Mr Bob McCreery, Cystic Fibrosis Association, 3567 East 49th Street, Cleveland, OH 44105, USA.

Vice Presidents: Général Yves Le Vacon, 55 Rue Lacordaire, Paris 75015, France.
Mr Alan Patrick, Coolbeg, Beaumont Drive, Ballintemple, Cork City, Ireland.

Treasurer: Mr Henk J. van Lier, c/o Amro Bank, P. O. Box 2059, 3500 GB Utrecht, The Netherlands.

Secretary: Mr Robert Johnson, 18 Scarsdale Villas, London W8 6PR, England.

World Health Organization Liaison Officer: Liliane Heidet, 124 Chemin de la Montagne, CH-1224 Chene-Bougeries, Switzerland.

MEMBERS OF THE ICF(M)A, 1985

Argentina

Dr O.H. Pivetta
President, Cystic Fibrosis Assoc. of Argentina
Beruti 2857 – 40. Piso "16", 1425 Buenos Aires, Argentina.

Australia

Mr Eric Ryan
National Secretary, Australian Cystic Fibrosis Federation Inc.
P. O. Box 225, Paddington, Queensland 4064, Australia.

Austria

Friedrich Komarek
President, Cystic Fibrosis Association
Heilisenkreuzerstr 29A, A 2384 Breitenfurt, Austria.

Brazil

Dr Ludma Trotta Dallalana
Assoc. Brazilara de Assistencia a Mucoviscidose
Av. Rui Barbosa, 716 Botafogo, Rio de Janeiro, Brazil.

Belgium

Mr Andre George
Secretary General, Association Belge de Lutte Contre la
Mucoviscidose
Place Georges Brugmann 29, 1060 Brussels, Belgium.

Canada

Mrs Cathleen Morrison
Executive Director, Canadian Cystic Fibrosis Foundation
586 Eglinton Avenue East, Suite 204, Toronto, Ontario M4P 1P2,
Canada.

Chile

Patricio Lira Venegas
Corporation Para La Fibrosis Quistica del Pancreas
La Canada 6506 (i), La Reina, Santiago, Chile.

Cuba

Dr Manuel Rojo Concepcion
President, Comision Cubana de Fibrosis Quistica
Servicio de Enfermedades Respr., Hospital Pediatrico Pedro
Borres, F entre 27 Y 29, Vedade Habana 4, La Habana, Cuba.

Czechoslovakia

Dr V. Vavrova
Cystic Fibrosis Association
Inst. Evolutionis Infantum Investigandae, 15112 Prague 5-Motol,
V Uvalu 84, Czechoslovakia.

Appendix 1

Denmark
Mrs Hanne Wendel Tyokjaer
Landsforeningen Til Bekaempelse af Cystisk Fibrose
Hyrdebakken 246, DK-8800 Viborg, Denmark.

Egypt
Dr Ekram Abdel-Salam
111 Abdel Aziz Suaoud Str., Manial, Cairo, Egypt.

Eire
Mr Ken French
Honorary Secretary, Cystic Fibrosis Association of Ireland
24, Lower Rathmines Road, Dublin 6, Eire.

Federal Republic of Germany
Mr Wolfgang Hutzler
Deutsche Gesellschaft zur Bekampfung der Mucoviscidose e.v.
Erlangen
Hainstrasse 8, Postfach 1810, 8500 Nürnberg, Federal Republic of
Germany

France
Mr Rene Barau
Administrator, Association Francaise de Lutte Contre la
Mucoviscidose
66 Boulevard St. Michel, 75 Paris 6e, France.

German Democratic Republic
Professor H. Dietzsch
Arbeitsgruppe zur Bekampfung der Mucoviscidose,
Fetcherstrasse 74, 8019 Dresden, German Democratic Republic.

Greece
Hellenic Cystic Fibrosis Association
Ag. Sikelianou 8, N. Psychico 15452, Athens, Greece.

Iceland

Dr H. Bergsteinsson
Icelandic Cystic Fibrosis Group
Barnaspitali Hringsins, Landspitalinn u/Baronsstig, Reykjavik-Postholf 101, Iceland.

Israel

Dr Nathan Durst
Cystic Fibrosis Foundation of Israel
Benjaminstr 5, P. O. Box 31171, Tel-Aviv 61311, Israel.

Italy

Diego Bortolusso
Secretary, Assoc. Italiana per la Contro la Fibrosi Cistica
Via Seminario n. 10, 30026 Portogruaro, Venezia, Italy.

Jordan

Cystic Fibrosis Jordan
University of Jordan, P. O. Box 13350, Amman, Jordan.

Mexico

Mr Antonio Gutierrez Cortina
President, Assoc. Mexicana de Fibrosis Quistica
Av. Revolucion 1389, 01040 Mexico D.F.

The Netherlands

Mr H. J. van Lier
Nederlandse Cystic Fibrosis Stichting
c/o Amro Bank, P. O. Box 2059, 3500 Utrecht, The Netherlands.

New Zealand

Mr C. W. McDonald
National Secretary, Cystic Fibrosis Association of New Zealand
P. O. Box 1755, Wellington, New Zealand.

Norway

Dr Per Espeli
Norwegian Cystic Fibrosis Association
c/o Norges Handikapforbund, Nils Hansensvei 2, Oslo 6, Norway.

Appendix 1

Poland

Professor Krystyna Boskova
Polish Cystic Fibrosis Association
National Institute of Mother and Child, Ul Kasprzaka, 17,
Warsaw, Poland.

South Africa

Mrs M. E. Kay
Southern Africa Cystic Fibrosis Association
Addington Hospital, Durban, Natal, South Africa.

Spain

Dr Jeronimo Pujol, President
Asociacion Espanola Contra la Fibrosis Quistica
Avda. S. Antonio M. Claret 167, Barcelona 25, Spain.

Sweden

Miss Birgitta Carlson
Riskforeningen for Cystisk Fibros
Box 3049, 750 03 Uppsala, Sweden.

Switzerland

Mr H. Muller
Secretary, Swiss Cystic Fibrosis Association
Bellevuestrasse 166, P. O. Box 24, CH-3028 Spiegel/BE, Switzerland.

Turkey

Dr Omar Ozalp
Department of Pediatrics, University of Hacettepe, Ankara,
Turkey.

Uruguay

Dr Carlos Boccoleri
Cystic Fibrosis Association of Uruguay
Br. Artigas 1465 esq. Palmer, Montevideo, Uruguay.

UK

Mrs Barbara Bentley
Cystic Fibrosis Research Trust
5, Blyth Road, Bromley, Kent BR1 3BS, UK.

Association of CF Adults (UK),
288 New Road, Ferndown,
Dorset BH22 8EP, UK.

USA

Robert K. Dresing Esq.
President,
Cystic Fibrosis Foundation,
6000 Executive Boulevard, Suite 510, Rockville, Maryland 20852,
USA.

Yugoslavia

Dr Streten Sicevic
Cystic Fibrosis Association of Yugoslavia
Mother and Child Institute of Serbia, 8, Radoja Dakica Street,
11071 New Belgrade, Yugoslavia.

ASSOCIATE MEMBERS OF THE ICF(M)A

Finland

Mr Ilpo Vilkkumaa
Cystic Fibrosis Association of Finland
Keuhkovammaliitto, Pohjoinen Hesperiankatu 15 A,
00260 Helsinki 26, Finland.

Hungary

Dr Kalman Gyurkovits
N. W. G. for Cystic Fibrosis
Medical University School of Szeged, Koranyi Fasor 18, H-6701,
Szeged, P. O. Box 471, Hungary

Appendix 1

India

Bhulabhai D. Patel, M.D.
82-B Embassy Apartments, 46 Nepean Sea Road, Bombay 36, India.

Portugal

Dr A. Valido
Rua Manuel Faria de Sousa No 16, Santo Amaro de Oeiras, 2780 Oeiras, Portugal.

USSR

Professor Sergei V. Rachinsky, M.D.
Head of Dept. of Pulmonology, Institute of Paediatrics, Academy of Medical Sciences of the USSR, V-292 Lomonosovsky PR 2, Moscow, USSR.

Dr Vladimir K. Tatochenko
Institute of Paediatrics
Academy of Medical Sciences of the USSR, V-292 Lomonosovsky PR 2, Moscow, USSR.

APPENDIX 2

Glossary

Acidosis — Condition resulting from accumulation of acid or depletion of the alkaline (bicarbonate) reserves in the blood or body tissues.

Aerosols — Medications given by inhalation, usually involving the wearing of a mask over the nose and mouth. In CF antibiotics, bronchodilators, saline, and occasionally mucolytics are given this way.

Alleles — The two forms of the same gene coexisting in the same cell, one being inherited from each of the parents.

Alveolae — Tiny, air-filled sacs in the lung tissue.

Antibody — The product of the body's immunological response to a foreign antigen, which specifically inactivates that antigen.

Antigen — A protein or other molecule foreign to the body, which can produce an immunological response in an animal challenged by it.

Autosome — All chromosomes other than the sex chromosomes.

Bacteria — Microorganisms (e.g. staphylococci, pseudomonas), some of which may invade healthy tissues, others only damaged tissue, to cause infections. Some bacteria, e.g. the *Bacillus coli* of the large bowel, cause no infection and are in fact necessary for health.

Ball-valve effects — These occur in those segments of the lung that have become overdistended through air getting past an obstruction on breathing in, but less getting past on breathing out.

Base — A substance that reacts with an acid to form a salt and water only.

Bronchiectasis — A state of permanent weakening of the bronchial walls, often because of infections and ball-valve phenomena which result in poor drainage of infected mucus.

Bronchioles — Small bronchi.

126

Appendix 2

Bronchodilator — A substance capable of relieving bronchospasm.

Bronchospasm — A reversible spasm (contraction) of the bronchi.

Bronchus (plural **Bronchi**) — Major branch of the airways.

Carrier — An individual who has inherited a particular defective form of a recessive gene from one of his parents, but a normal form from the other. He thus 'carries' the defective gene, but suffers no ill effects from it.

Cholecystitis — Inflammation of the gall bladder, often associated with gallstones.

Chromosomes — The structures within each cell that contain the genetic material.

Cilia — Minute mobile, hair-like processes projecting from the outer surface of a cell. The airways are lined with ciliated cells.

Ciliary dyskinesis factor — A substance able to disrupt synchronized movement of cilia.

Cirrhosis — Fibrosis of the liver, interfering with the passage of blood from the intestine through liver cells.

Coeliac disease — An inability to digest wheat proteins.

Consanguinity — Inbreeding between genetically related members of the same family.

Diploid — Cells carrying two sets of genetic information.

DNA (Deoxyribonucleic acid) — The major component of the genetic material. The biological molecule that codes for all the information needed to construct a human being from a single fertilized egg.

Dominant — An abnormal gene, the effects of which are not masked by the presence of its normal counterpart in the same cell.

Duodenal intubation — A process whereby the end of a soft polythene tube is swallowed and passed via the stomach into the duodenum, allowing the contents to be studied chemically, both as regards enzymes and alkalinity.

Endocrine glands — These pass their secretions directly into the bloodstream, e.g. insulin and glucagon from the pancreas.

Emphysema — Permanent overdistention of the alveolae in the lung.

Enema — Injection of liquid into the rectum.

Cystic Fibrosis: the facts

Exocrine gland — A gland that passes its secretions by ducts, e.g. trypsin and lipase from the pancreas. (The pancreas is both an exocrine and an endocrine gland.)

Fibroblasts — A very common cell type found in many tissues of the body and readily grown in culture.

Fibrosis — The replacement of normal tissue with scar tissue, e.g. in the pancreas. Hence the name *Cystic Fibrosis*: fluid-filled cysts develop in the obstructed parts of the pancreas.

Flatus — Breaking of wind.

Genes — Coding regions of DNA.

Genome — All the genetic information of an individual.

Glycoproteins — Large, complex biological molecules consisting of carbohydrate units attached to a protein backbone.

Haematemesis — The vomiting of blood. In CF this would most often be associated with cirrhosis and varices.

Haemoptysis — The coughing of blood, usually indicative of advanced CF.

Haploid — Cells carrying one set of genetic information (i.e. eggs and sperm).

Heterozygote — An individual who has inherited different forms of a particular gene from both parents.

Homozygote — An individual who has inherited identical forms of a particular gene from both parents.

Ileus — Literally, a disorder of motility of the ileum, resulting in the contents not being propelled towards the colon. In meconium ileus, contents are not propelled because of the tenacious meconium.

Ileostomy — The bringing of a loop of ileum to open onto the anterior abdominal wall to allow bowel contents to be passed, when there is an obstruction lower down.

Intussusception — A pathological process when a section of the small intestine closer to the stomach folds into the adjoining region of downstream bowel, endangering its blood supply.

Ion — An electrically charged atom or molecule.

Isotonic — Having the same electrolytic composition, as do most body tissues.

Lingula — Part of the upper lobe of the left lung.

Leukocytes — White blood cells.

Malabsorption — Inability to absorb food normally in intestines due to poor digestion.

MCT oil — Oil containing medium-chain triglycerides. These can be absorbed directly into the bloodstream from the intestine.

Meconium — The first dark-green stools of the newborn.

Meconium ileus — An obstruction of the small intestine at birth.

Meiosis — The cell division process by which haploid cells are made from diploid ones.

Mesentery — The membrane carrying the blood vessels to and from the bowel.

Messenger RNA — Copied from DNA by transcription, this molecule is the blueprint for translation of the genetic information into biologically useful molecules, proteins.

Mucolytic — Substance capable of thinning mucus. It may do this by increasing the water content of the mucus or by breaking chemical bonds between sulphur and hydrogen.

Mutation — The occurrence of a spontaneous abnormality in a gene that is not found in the genes of the parent's cells.

Nasal polyp — A growth resulting from the heaping up of mucous membrane in the nostril. Common in older children with CF.

Non-polar — A molecule that does not contain an electric dipole (*see* Polar).

Osteomyelitis — Infection of the bone, often caused by *Staphylococcus* bacteria, generally in people free of CF.

Pancreatin — Extract of animal pancreas.

Parenteral — Given by a route other than the alimentary canal (digestive system) – usually by vein.

Pathogenesis — The evolution of the abnormal (pathological) changes of a disease process.

Peritoneum — The membrane lining the walls of the abdomen.

Peritonitis — An acute inflammation of the peritoneum.

Pneumothorax — Air trapped between the outside (pleural) surface of the lung and the chest wall. This splints the lung and prevents its normal movement during breathing. In CF it would occur with the rupture of overdistended (emphysematous) alveoli. Removal of the air by a needle attached to an underwater drain may be necessary.

Polar Molecule — A molecule containing two equal point electric charges of opposite sign (a dipole) separated by a small distance.

Probe — A segment of DNA that is complementary to part or all of the DNA sequence of interest.

Prolapsed rectum — Found in young infants with CF, usually before diagnosis. Malabsorption of fat, with very frequent stools, results in the inner lining of the rectum protruding through the anus.

Proximal bowel — Section of bowel closer to the mouth. (**Distal bowel** — Bowel section further from mouth, i.e. closer to anus.)

Recessive — An abnormal gene, the effects of which are masked by the presence of its normal counterpart in the same cell.

Recombination — The physical process by which new combinations of genes are made by shuffling of the genetic information prior to cell division.

Sclerosing agents — Drugs that strengthen the blood vessel wall.

Spirometer — An instrument for measuring the air breathed into and out of the lungs.

Sputum — Phlegm coughed up from the airway passages.

Steatorrhoea — Literally, fatty diarrhoea. Recognized by pale, bulky, foul-smelling stools.

Thalassaemia — An inherited disease caused by abnormalities in the haemoglobin of the blood.

Varices — Dilated veins.

X-linked — A gene on the X chromosome.

Index

131

Index

Index

screening 36
secretions 96–8
sex chromosome 66
Shwachman score 43–6
sodium 97, 101
spirometer 42
Staphylococcus aureus 11, 18, 48, 50
starch 22
steatorrhoea 10, 11, 25, 28
sugars 20, 22
sweat 32, 97
sweat gland 32
sweat test 34, 35

thalassaemia 81, 107

The Cystic Fibrosis Research
 Trust 114, 115
tissue culture 101–5
trace elements 61
trachea 15
trypsin 23, 59

ultrasound 86, 87

varices 62
vitamins 61

X-linked 109